Hot Times

How to Eat Well, Live Healthy,
and Feel Sexy During the Change

A REVISED AND UPDATED EDITION
OF *Super Nutrition for Menopause*

Ann Louise Gittleman, Ph.D., CNS

AVERY

a member of Penguin Group (USA) Inc.

New York

AVERY

Published by the Penguin Group • Penguin Group (USA) Inc., 375 Hudson Street,
New York, New York 10014, USA • Penguin Group (Canada), 90 Eglinton Avenue East, Suite 700, Toronto,
Ontario M4P 2Y3, Canada (a division of Pearson Penguin Canada Inc.) • Penguin Books Ltd, 80 Strand,
London WC2R 0RL, England • Penguin Ireland, 25 St Stephen's Green, Dublin 2, Ireland (a division of
Penguin Books Ltd) • Penguin Group (Australia), 250 Camberwell Road, Camberwell, Victoria 3124, Australia
(a division of Pearson Australia Group Pty Ltd) • Penguin Books India Pvt Ltd, 11 Community Centre,
Panchsheel Park, New Delhi–110 017, India • Penguin Group (NZ), Cnr Airborne and Rosedale Roads,
Albany, Auckland 1310, New Zealand (a division of Pearson New Zealand Ltd) • Penguin Books
(South Africa) (Pty) Ltd, 24 Sturdee Avenue, Rosebank, Johannesburg 2196, South Africa

Penguin Books Ltd, Registered Offices:
80 Strand, London WC2R 0RL, England

Table 7-1 and the Hijiki Noodle recipe are reprinted from *Super Nutrition for Women*
(Bantam, 2004) and are used with permission.

Library of Congress Cataloging-in-Publication Data

Gittleman, Ann Louise.
Hot times : How to eat well, live healthy, and feel sexy during the change / Ann Louise Gittleman.—2nd ed.
p. cm.
First ed. published in 1993 under title: Super nutrition for menopause.
Includes bibliographical references and index.
ISBN 1-58333-214-6
1. Menopause.   2. Menopause—Nutritional aspects.   3. Middle-aged women—Health and hygiene.
I. Gittleman, Ann Louise. Super nutrition for menopause.   II. Title.

RG186.H7794   2005   2004066340
618.1'75—dc22

Printed in the United States of America
1   3   5   7   9   10   8   6   4   2

Book design by Stephanie Huntwork

Hot Times

ACKNOWLEDGMENTS

My thanks, first and foremost, to my readers and patients who have been such faithful followers for nearly twenty-five years. Thank you for the trust you have placed in me. I will always appreciate your support and loyalty. Rest assured, I will always strive for the truth and write from my heart.

Thank you to my agent, Suzanne Cohn, and the entire Avery team who have been so excited about this updated and revised edition of my book. Special thanks to publisher Megan Newman, whose passion and commitment to excellence are contagious. Kudos to my editor, Kristen Jennings, whose patience and diligence with this manuscript were most admirable. Thanks for everything, Kristen. To associate publisher Kate Stark, thanks for all of your unwavering support and marketing expertise. I am also grateful for the extraordinary "eagle eyes" of copy editor Antonia Rachiele.

My most sincere appreciation goes to J. Lynne Dodson for her literary assistance with my book.

Lynne, you are the "professional's professional" and I am so thankful for your sweet spirit and diligence. We have worked together for more than ten years and you have never failed to be there round-the-clock. And, I know you will all want to join me in acknowledging Linda Shapiro and Charli Sorenson for helping me create, tweak, and test-taste the culinary delights in this book. Many of the new recipes presented in this revised edition were inspired by other wonderful cooks, including Jamie Zayach, Diana Israel, Deborah Boschee, Laura Hitchman, Melissa Myers, and Elaine Friedman. I also wish to thank all of my readers and followers on the Forum and iVillage websites who have shared their recipes and tips. You will note, of course, that both the menus and the recipes reflect the carb-conscious eating style that is here to stay.

Sincere appreciation is extended to Stuart Gittleman, Operations and Business Manager of First Lady of Nutrition, Inc., for keeping up with my schedule during the writing of this book. Thanks, also, to Debbie Judd, R.N., who has been working with me side by side as my Outreach Coordinator for First Lady venues. Debbie is a doll and has a 24/7 work ethic that makes her just like "family" to Stuart and me. She also has a terrific husband, Dr. Mike, whose dry sense of humor contributes just the right dose of comic relief.

I also wish to thank my personal support system of *Hot Times* women: Coleen O'Shea; Nan Fuchs, Ph.D.; Hyla Cass, M.D.; Shirley Scott, M.D.; Elizabeth Krichman; Paula Breen; Linda Alexander; Linda Hooper; Sandra Gittleman; Shira Gittleman; Carol Templeton; Ellie Cullen; Frankie Boyer; Deborah Ray; Darlene Kvist; Lynn Gordon; Roon Frost; Connie Deans; Jo Len Schoor; Joanie Greggains; Kathie Moe; Julia Trick, N.D.; Carolyn Bartholomew; Lindsey Johnson; Denise Jones; Cheryl Siroshton; Diane Romeo, D.C.; Judi Wilson; Roz Livingston; and Myrna Rasmussen.

And to these *Hot Times* men: James Templeton (first and foremost, always); Joel Legard; Kyle Motley; Verne Hamilton; Joe Sharnetsky; Bob Monroe; Elson Haas, M.D.; Kinnie McCabe, M.D.; Len Kasten; Fred Pescatore, M.D.; Bill Sardi; Roy Speiser, D.C., Ph.D.; Jonny Bowden, M.S., CNS; Richard Fernandez; and Dickson Ward.

CONTENTS

It is with great pleasure that I write the foreword to a book that is destined to be a classic. I have admired the work of Ann Louise Gittleman for many years, and although neither of us would like to admit it, she was one of my earliest teachers. I recall interviewing her on the radio when I was first starting out in the field of nutritional medicine, when I would fill in for Dr. Robert Atkins on his radio show. I was terrified because she was so much more knowledgeable than I was and I did not want to appear stupid. So I read all her books and became even more impressed. She was one of the greats even way back then. She was someone I admired, and I still do. She continues to learn, explore, and best of all, get the message out to millions of adoring fans.

In my opinion, menopause and perimenopause have become too medicalized, and women have suffered because of that. Menopause should not be treated as if it were a disease. Unfortunately, that is how these incredible years in a woman's life are now being seen. Once it was realized how many women were about to enter these years, menopause was seen as a great growth opportunity for any pharmaceutical company who had the technology to produce hormones. What a great idea to be able to patent a technology and falsely claim that what you produced saved lives, preserved bones, protected people from heart disease, and decreased their risk for cancer. What would you say if that same product used by millions of women actually did the reverse of all those things? What would you say if there was a woman who could tell you how to take control of your life, and enjoy the vitality you're used to without any of the side effects, and you could do it all naturally? Ann Louise and *Hot Times* are just what you have been looking for.

With the advent of the landmark studies proving conventional hormone replacement therapy causes more harm than good, millions of women worldwide have been left in a very precarious position. If you are on hormonal replacement, do you discontinue those drugs? How can you treat your symptoms? Are there alternatives to hormone replacement therapy? Is there such a thing as natural or bioidentical hormones, and do they work? The answers to all of these most common concerns facing so many women today are now available in this breakthrough book.

It is possible to protect yourself and those around you from all the symptoms associated with premenstrual syndrome, perimenopause, and menopause itself when you can prepare your body. We have known for years that there are many biological elements that change during this time of a woman's life. The conventional medical way of thinking reflects only the most obvious decline—hormones—but there is so much more to it than this. Not only is there more to menopause than hormones, there is more to treatment than just estrogen and progesterone. Insulin, cortisol, and DHEA, to name a few of the many hormones your body secretes, are also crucial players in how your body reacts to these conditions. Your body must be prepared for the obvious changes, but also for the ones that no one has told you about—until now.

Although these other hormones are no less important, they have taken a back seat to the big ones. *Hot Times* will help you prepare your entire body for the change as you discover the importance of dietary habits such as decreasing the amount of sugar you eat, increasing the amount of healthy fats in your diet, cutting out damaging lifestyle habits such as caffeine and nicotine consumption, and getting the right amount of sleep.

The role of nutritional supplements also cannot be overlooked. These safe over-the-counter preparations have been used literally for centuries to help women handle their most common problems. Their safety and effectiveness have been well documented and clinically researched and should be a part of every woman's daily regimen. There is more to being a woman than just taking calcium. Vitamins, minerals, and essential fatty acids play a crucial role in health and must be embraced during these hot times.

Women are the primary health care consumers and providers in North America and Europe. They are more willing to try novel approaches, especially if these methods are safe. If menopause happened to men, you can rest assured that we'd have more answers than we currently possess. However, no one has more answers to the problems associated with this great change than Ann Louise. She was there before anyone else—before menopause was trendy. She has worked with thousands of clients and helped hundreds of thousands more through her books, newsletters, and lectures. I know she can help you through this transformational time of your life, and I am sure you will love this book as much as I have and make it a part of your permanent collection.

FRED PESCATORE, M.D., author of *The Hamptons Diet*

Introduction

Today, between 55 and 70 million American women are menopausal, and our ranks are increasing at a rate of about 4,200 a day. That's nearly three a minute! Our great advantage as we approach this often challenging phase in our health and development is that, unlike previous generations, we are the beneficiaries of past decades of increasingly frank discussions of sexuality and health; an unprecedented availability of information via the Internet; discoveries in genetics, molecular biology, and computer-assisted diagnosis; and the institutional changes that have happened as a result of all these factors.

For example, it's only been within the past fifteen years or so that many in the medical establishment acknowledged what women have known all along—we are different from men. Not just in the obvious senses, but in some very fundamental ways that affect both the way illnesses develop and how they should be treated. Take heart disease, for example. For decades, it has been viewed medically as primarily a male disease. Major research studies begun in the 1940s focused on men, and the diagnostic tools and treatments that resulted were based on the disease's progress in men. Yet we now know heart disease is the number-one killer of women. And unlike a man's, a woman's symptoms are usually more subtle, and blockages tend to develop in smaller vessels, making missed diagnoses common. Also, women fail to recover as quickly as men, and their survival after bypass surgery is less certain.

In 1994, the U.S. Food and Drug Administration (FDA) acknowledged the importance of investigating the unique field of women's health when it established the Office of Women's Health. Its mandate is to fund research focused on health issues vital to women. At about the same time, the federal government stipulated that studies funded with grants from the National Institutes of Health must include women in their patient base and/or evaluate the impact of their findings on women's health. Perhaps no topic has benefited from this focused research more than that of hormone replacement therapy (HRT).

WOMEN AND HORMONES: PAST, PRESENT, AND FUTURE

In the 1950s, most women who asked for help with symptoms like hot flashes and vaginal dryness were told that the condition was "all in their heads." In the mid-1960s, the landmark book *Feminine Forever*, by Robert A. Wilson, M.D., a New York gynecologist, introduced the estrogen deficiency theory. Wilson, no doubt inspired by monies received from drug companies, believed that estrogen was the panacea that could cure any and every menopausal symptom. Wilson contended that without estrogen at menopause, all women are destined to become sexless "caricatures of their former selves . . . the equivalent of eunuch[s]." In the early 1970s, physicians were routinely dispensing both estrogen and tranquilizers; the combination was probably not only for menopause but also for the trauma resulting from Robert Wilson's book.

In the mid-1970s, however, research studies began to link the use of estrogen in postmenopausal women to rate increases in cancer of the uterus, and as a result, the hormone's use declined for several years. Then, when newer studies showed that the addition of a synthetic form of progesterone known as progestin could protect women against uterine cancer, postmenopausal hormone therapy once again became the answer. Even with the documented dangers, by 1990, over 10 million American women were on HRT.

But thankfully, that has now come to a screeching halt. In 2002, the Women's Health Initiative's (WHI) long-term study of the effects of HRT on cardiovascular disease in women was shut down three years early when it was discovered that long-term use of HRT increased a woman's risk of stroke by 41 percent, heart attack by 29 percent, and breast cancer by 24 percent. Less than a year later, another WHI study of the effects of HRT on memory reported that older women on HRT had twice the risk of developing dementia. In Britain, at about the same time, the Million Women Study was halted when results indicated an increased risk of breast cancer and its severity among women taking hormone replacement therapy. Finally, in 2004, a Swedish study of menopausal breast cancer survivors on HRT was halted because of an unacceptably high risk of breast cancer recurrence.

The medicalization of menopause has not worked. Women need, deserve, and are beginning to insist on a way to regain their lives that is free from hot flashes, sexual decline, and insomnia and that doesn't involve life-threatening side effects.

A NEW PERSPECTIVE
ON MENOPAUSE

Menopause is big business, and we menopausal women have become a prime target market. Unfortunately, the health problems that become a greater risk for women at menopause—heart disease, cancer, and osteoporosis—are being linked solely to menopause. This narrow view discounts numerous biochemical, dietary, and lifestyle factors that have been in play for many years of a woman's life, long before menopause, leaving many a female body totally out of balance. This view also disempowers us, implying that we have no control over what is happening to our bodies. But we know better.

Understanding Your Body

What happens at menopause is explained by the word *menopause* itself. Coming from the Greek, *men pausis,* menopause literally means "month to end," relating to the final monthly menstrual period. The term *menopause* is oftentimes used interchangeably with the more precise term *climacteric.* The climacteric is the hormonal changes that start occurring in a woman's body from about the age of 35 and continue to the age of approximately 50. The ovaries, in the course of this natural cycle, dramatically decrease production of the female hormones estrogen and progesterone.

While much attention has been given to the role of estrogen deficiency during menopause, the importance of progesterone is often overlooked. Progesterone is one of the body's most important hormones, known for its ability to maintain pregnancy. But it also has benefits far beyond its role in menstrual cycles and pregnancy, and lack of this essential hormone affects many of our body systems. By making sure our progesterone levels are adequate, we can avoid many of the symptoms of menopause and aging.

A fact that also needs to be considered is that menopause occurs when the effects of the natural biological aging process are beginning to appear. As we grow older, our bodies do not work the way they did earlier in life, and our poor dietary and lifestyle habits begin to take a heavier toll. This time of life is also often filled with stressful changes for many women: we may find ourselves parenting our parents as they age; our children, who have left home, may be returning home with their children; and many women at this age find themselves single, either through the death of a spouse or divorce.

The uncomfortable symptoms associated with menopause—such as hot flashes, vaginal dryness, and mood swings—are connected to the lowered hormonal output common in women in this time of life, but they are not experienced by all women. The more serious health concerns at midlife are also not experienced by all women. So menopause, while occurring universally, is still very much a personal matter.

After studying the accepted medical, psychological, social, and emotional beliefs on menopause, I came to three major conclusions about the medical community's current perceptions:

1. Almost without exception, every health problem experienced by women in midlife is somehow blamed on the natural hormonal changes that take place during menopause.
2. There is a common misconception that menopause is a pathological process and that the problems associated with it (hot flashes, sexual decline, osteoporosis, heart disease) are inevitable without medical intervention.
3. The cumulative effects of long-term nutrient deficiencies and negative lifestyle habits—which begin in our teens and continue through our 40s—have been blatantly ignored.

As you read on, you will see that many of these misconceptions are dispelled. In their place, you will come to a new understanding of menopause as one of the greatest milestones in a woman's lifecycle—one that can be managed with the right diet and lifestyle strategies, without medication.

NUTRITION AND MENOPAUSE

It is a little-known fact that during menopause, the reduced amount of estrogen and progesterone from the ovaries is naturally compensated for by hormones produced elsewhere in the body, primarily the adrenal glands and body fat, nature's backup system. When our bodies are overstressed, our adrenals can become exhausted, and this natural backup system can fail, leaving us unprotected and making menopause far more difficult than Mother Nature intended it to be. Because progesterone is necessary for the production of adrenal hormones, when the adrenals are overworked and the hormones they produce are depleted, progesterone is constantly used to replenish the system. This stress on our adrenals may leave many of us with progesterone deficiency, which can cause bone loss, thinning hair, and facial whiskers. An imbalance of the progesterone/estrogen levels creates a condition called unopposed estrogen dominance, and excessive amounts of estrogen in the body lead to increased incidence of breast cancer, bone loss, and hypothyroidism.

This lack of progesterone is particularly common five to eight years before menopause, because many of us no longer ovulate. But this process does not occur in all women. While about 75 percent of us experience distressing symptoms purportedly connected to declining estrogen and progesterone, the remaining 25 percent do not suffer any adverse effects. Why? Because for that 25 percent of women, their adrenal system functions properly and they are able to maintain an appropriate balance of hormones. What is their secret weapon? The answer is simple—proper nutrition and a healthy lifestyle.

For too many of us, poor nutritional and lifestyle habits create an unbalanced body chemistry, which is a potent underlying cause of menopausal woes. Dietary habits carried to excess, such as consuming too much sugar and caffeine and following strict fat-free diets, stress our bodies. For example, caffeine stimulates the adrenal glands, causing adrenaline to be released into the bloodstream. Adrenaline activates our fight-or-flight response, increasing our heart rate, blood pressure, and blood sugar level. When this initial rush wears off, blood sugar drops to lower levels than before the coffee was consumed and leaves the adrenal glands in a depleted state. And then it's time for another cup of coffee. Add sugar and the problem is intensified, because refined sugars have the same stressful effect on the adrenal glands. In a single day in the United States alone, over 330 million cups of coffee are consumed.

Our excessive dietary habits not only lead to adrenal exhaustion that results in damage to our backup system, they also contribute to other, more serious health problems as we enter our middle years. Studies show that women between the ages of 34 and 59 who drink four or more cups of coffee a day have an incidence of hip fractures almost three times greater than do women who drink little or none at all. And what about soft drinks? We Americans consume more than 52 gallons per person per year, and the phosphates contained in that fizzy sugar water play havoc with calcium absorption. The past popularity of the no- to low-fat diets and the consumption of the wrong kinds of fats—particularly processed oils and hydrogenated fats like margarine and vegetable shortening—have led to a nationwide deficiency of the essential fatty acids. Yet, it's those essential fats that make calcium available for the tissues and elevate calcium levels in the bloodstream.

And lifestyle habits can't be ignored. Smoking cigarettes, drinking alcohol, getting too little exercise, and too much stress add to the midlife woman's health problems. Ignoring these lifestyle and dietary factors and focusing on estrogen as the only deficiency is unsound and bad medicine.

Unfortunately, even when we've been made aware of the nutritional impact on disease, the information available has been too simplistic or not comprehensive enough to actually help us. We've heard for years that calcium is the singular mineral that builds strong bones and teeth, and that inadequate calcium levels lead to osteoporosis. So we drink our milk and believe we're protected. But actually, the latest research suggests that it's not calcium but its overshadowed counterpart, the mineral magnesium, that is the key ingredient for not only strong bones but also healthy hearts. By consuming too many high-calcium dairy products, we are actually interfering with magnesium absorption and creating blockages in our blood vessels. Recent nutritional research also links magnesium deficiencies to a host of conditions that begin to surface in women at midlife, such as cardiovascular disease, depression, and osteoporosis.

Finding a Nutritional Solution

While serving as the director of nutrition at the Pritikin Longevity Center in Santa Monica, California, I saw how dramatic changes in health took place in patients with heart disease, diabetes, and hypertension once they followed a suitable diet and exercise program. After leaving Pritikin for my own practice, I worked with countless women, reviewing thousands of diet histories. I developed diet and supplement programs for allergies, weight loss, weight gain, eating disorders, irritable bowel syndrome, parasites, PMS, and yeast infections. Time and time again, I saw how good nutrition and the right supplements could prevent, control, and cure these disorders. Why not a nutrition program to prevent or control the unpleasant symptoms associated with a natural life change like menopause?

Our health at midlife has its roots in our teens, 20s, and 30s. It is during these decades that we need to start taking in enough bone-building minerals, getting enough proper and consistent exercise, and developing positive lifestyle and dietary habits. Without proper nutritional reinforcement throughout life, the major glandular changes that take place in our 40s and 50s can become medical crises rather than natural transitions. At midlife, hormone levels fluctuate, creating imbalances in calcium, magnesium, and a number of other important minerals and vitamins needed for good health. If imbalances already exist as the result of a lifetime of nutritional neglect, they become magnified by the dramatic glandular changes taking place at menopause. Illnesses like diabetes, hypertension, heart disease, and osteoporosis become greater risks as time passes.

But the problems we associate with menopause are not inevitable. Even if we have been neglectful in the past, the uncomfortable symptoms of menopause can become a wake-up call, alerting us to take charge of our own health. Menopause can be a positive motivational factor to make the dietary and lifestyle changes that will not only ease our passage through menopause but also benefit our health for the rest of our lives. A diet of unprocessed, unrefined, natural foods—including green leafy vegetables, fresh fruits, whole grains, fish, poultry, lean meat, nuts, seeds, and legumes, and moderate amounts of natural and unprocessed oils—paves the way to good health.

We can have a great deal of control over how we will respond to menopause by preparing early. Taking an inventory of our eating habits, weight, exercise patterns, smoking and drinking history, and heredity factors before menopause occurs will give us some substantial clues to our own journey through this passage. Every woman's menopause experience is different, based on these lifestyle and heredity factors. Up to menopause, balanced hormones provide us with additional protection against heart disease and osteoporosis. After menopause, we are on our own, and the foundation we have laid and our current bad habits make their consequences known.

TAKE CHARGE OF YOUR MENOPAUSE TREATMENT NOW

On a more positive note, premenopausal clinics are springing up all over the country. These clinics focus on women in their mid-30s and mid-40s, when estrogen levels first begin to decline, and use a number of screening tools and medical tests to assess a woman's risk of heart disease, osteoporosis, and cancer (cervical, uterine, ovarian, breast), as well as postmenopausal urinary incontinence. By taking advantage of the diagnostic and assessment procedures these clinics have to offer, we can head off potential difficulties. The earlier we take the time to reevaluate our lifestyles and make meaningful changes, the better our midlife years will be.

Medical attitudes are changing, and an increasing number of physicians are incorporating nutritional and alternative therapies into their practices. Nevertheless, your health is ultimately up to you.

Become informed about menopause and the aging process. Reading this book will get you off to a good start. Many popular magazines readily available at your neighborhood grocery store offer a wealth of additional information, and the Internet puts information from all over the world onto your desktop instantly.

Ask your doctor about nutrition and other alternative treatments when he or she pulls out the prescription pad. (Traditionally trained physicians are woefully ignorant of nutritional principles, so you may need to guide this discussion.) When you ask questions of your health care provider, don't settle for less-than-satisfactory answers. You need to know why a test is being recommended, what it should show, and what will happen once results are in. You need to know what the side effects are of a drug being prescribed, if natural alternatives are available, and what happens if the drug fails. Be skeptical. There is still a great deal medical science doesn't know, especially about the intricate workings of our hormones. Be wary of a doctor who refuses to give any alternatives or who never admits to not knowing the answer. Not all your questions can be answered.

You should also be open to getting a second opinion. The Resource list at the back of this book offers several referral sources to naturopathic and holistic providers, who may present nonmedicated or noninvasive options. Look for another health care provider if yours is unwilling to give you the time you need to have your questions answered, doesn't listen to your concerns or suggestions, or fails to give you or your symptoms the respect you and they deserve.

Above all, listen to your body. For too long, women allowed physicians to convince them their symptoms were "all in their head." Some women are alive today because they refused to let the vagueness of their symptoms justify a lack of effort to diagnose and treat their heart disease.

HOT TIMES WOMEN

As far as I am concerned, we are all Hot Times women. Not only are the menopausal years a time when we endure "power" surges (otherwise known as hot flashes) and other changes in our bodies, they are also a time when many of us truly come into our own. I encourage you to use this book as a guide to all of your Hot Times concerns. Whether you need to know how to use nutritional remedies to address symptoms of hot flashes, night sweats, tissue dryness, lack of libido, sleeplessness, and mood swings or to deal with stress, osteoporosis, heart disease, diabetes, breast cancer, or hypothyroidism, this book has answers for you. The Hot Times Diet, in Chapter 7, and the menus and recipes, in Chapter 8, provide a practical, proactive, and protective outlet for all the key dietary recommendations addressed throughout the previous chapters.

It is my hope that this book will empower women, from adolescence to the Hot Times transition, to continue the nutritional revolution that has changed the way in which we view and treat menopause. Attention to proper diet, exercise, lifestyle changes, and what the body is saying will make the journey into midlife a time of great freedom and renewed energy. The postmenopausal years should be the best time of a woman's life, when she is freed of child-rearing responsibilities and rewarded with good health. As Margaret Mead put it, "The most creative force in the world is the menopausal woman with zest." Keeping our bodies in biochemical balance is a lifetime adventure that will assure that our passage through each stage of life is filled with zest. The time to prepare is now.

ONE

Menopause: Get Control of Your Symptoms

HOT FLASHES, SEXUAL CHANGES, SLEEPLESSNESS, DEPRES-
sion, and weight gain are the focus of this chapter. But these symptoms don't just happen overnight. Actually, menopause, or the end
of your monthly periods, is a natural transition that occurs over a period of about fifteen years, from approximately 35 to 50 years of age.
This time frame, known as the climacteric, is characterized by fluctuating hormone levels. The production of estrogen and progesterone
by your ovaries diminishes gradually until your monthly periods completely stop.

The average age of menopause for American women is 51. Because heredity plays a significant role, the best predictor of when you
will reach menopause is the age at which your mother went through
it. But there are many factors based on heredity, environment, and
body type that can provide an indicator of when you may go through
menopause. If you are black or if you can trace your family roots to
southern Europe or the Mediterranean, you will probably experience
menopause earlier. Female athletes (especially marathon runners),
extremely thin women like fashion models, and women with eating
disorders such as bulimia and anorexia are likely to experience earlier

menopause because of lack of body fat and low cholesterol levels. Later-occurring menopause is more common among white women of northern European origin. Women living in poor socioeconomic conditions reach menopause earlier than those with higher standards of living, but women who bear children after age 40 experience a later menopause.

Researchers tell us that if you are a smoker, you can reach an even earlier menopause—by three to four years. Egg production stops prematurely as a result of the damage nicotine and carbon monoxide inflict on the ovaries. If you are a strict vegetarian or have lower-than-normal cholesterol levels, you'll probably experience menopause earlier than the average. Other factors contributing to early menopause include having borne no children, being overweight, and having had a late puberty. If you have had your ovaries removed surgically and are not treated with hormone-replacement therapy, you are considered menopausal no matter what your age. Diseases of the pituitary gland and medical irradiation of the ovaries can also induce early menopause.

A CULTURAL PERSPECTIVE

Your experience of menopause is heavily influenced by the culture in which you live. As Western cultures until now have emphasized youth, beauty, and sexuality as ultimate female standards, it's no wonder that menopause is perceived as a time of loss and regret. Many women suffer needless depression at its approach. In non-Western cultures, on the other hand, menopause is viewed much differently. The cessation of childbearing is a positive event in a woman's life, and less attention is focused on physical discomforts. Women reaching menopause are regarded as having reached their peak of power. They are looked on as elders, full of wisdom and experience. Women in certain Native American tribes, for example, gained entry into the Grandmothers' Lodge upon reaching menopause. They were respected for the wisdom and power they attained by not losing their "wise blood." Where other cultures make menopause a rite of passage, our culture turns it into a medical event. We get caught up in focusing on "symptoms," and our lives often become a matter of "surviving" menopause.

Women today are changing all that—and it's about time. Coming of age during the sexual revolution of the 1970s, we are more open than our mothers were to discussing issues of sexuality, reproductive health, and overall health and well-being. New attitudes within the medical establishment are leading to major studies, such as the Women's Health Initiative of the National Institutes of Health.

"When a woman reaches age 50, she typically has another 30 years to live," Isaac Schiff, M.D., chief of obstetrics and gynecology at Massachusetts General Hospital, has been quoted as saying. "As physicians, we became interested not only in the quantity of her life, but the quality of it." Empowered by the wealth of information available on the Internet, from alternative practitioners, and via the women-focused research studies, you and I are likely to change forever the way this life stage is viewed in Western culture. At the same time, we will be able to support the major glandular changes that take place through the right diet, nutritional supplements, herbs, homeopathic remedies, exercise, and a positive attitude about ourselves. These effective methods of self-care, which I have organized into the Hot Times approach, will surely gift all of us with a renewed sense of freedom and energy so that we can take full advantage of the opportunities that await us in the years ahead.

UNDERSTANDING AND TREATING YOUR MENOPAUSAL SYMPTOMS

If I were to sit with five midlife women at a table and ask them about their menopause experience, I'd probably hear five different descriptions. Most women define menopause by their symptoms, but these can vary greatly from woman to woman. Sometimes women will notice two to three years of irregularity in their menstrual cycle, like changes in blood flow and frequency of the monthly period itself. The period may even suddenly go away for months at a time, then reappear. This is why most authorities suggest practicing birth control for at least a year after the last full period.

Other signals of approaching menopause include hot flashes and night sweats, vaginal dryness, urinary incontinence, headaches, irritability, insomnia, mood changes, changes in body weight, and loss of sexual drive and interest. Two other hormonally based changes include body-shape changes and altered perception of touch (see page 27). After menopause, some women may also experience shrinking breasts, thinning hair, and the appearance of facial whiskers due to the loss of progesterone.

The variation in symptoms among menopausal women may be explained by hormone imbalances caused by the delicate interrelation of hormones within the body. Estrogen and progesterone are part of the complex family of sex steroid hormones, which includes testosterone, cortisol, and DHEA (dehydroepiandrosterone). These are all made from cholesterol and work together to affect everything from your immune response to your libido. Estrogen itself is not a single hormone, but an entire class, including estradiol, estrone, and estriol. Estradiol is the dominant estrogen in premenopausal women. Estrone, which is produced from hormones stored in body fat, predominates in most postmenopausal women. It acts much like estradiol, but with less strength. Estriol, the weakest of these estrogens, is primarily found in pregnant women.

Sex steroids are made predominantly in the ovaries (and testes in men) and the adrenal glands, but can also be made in the brain, liver, and skin. The hormones are chemically very similar to one another and share the property that each can be converted into one or more of the others when a deficiency occurs. At menopause, for example, when your ovaries cease production of estradiol, your body can transform testosterone stored in your fat cells into estrone. Because of this interrelationship, supplementing one hormone without ensuring adequate levels of the others will probably create a hormonal imbalance.

These hormonal imbalances bring on a wide range of symptoms, as I describe throughout this book. Several hormones may bring on similar symptoms; for example, deficiencies in estrogen, progesterone, or DHEA are all associated with mood swings. Estrogen deficiency is associated with everything from hot flashes to depression. On the other hand, excess estrogen can lower your sex drive and cause you to gain weight and crave sweets. Too little or too much of these steroid hormones is associated with asthma, anorexia, high blood pressure, osteoporosis, and sleep disorders.

Get to Know Your Hormones

You may experience enough of these changes to recognize the start of your menopause. On the other hand, you may be among the approximately 20 percent of women who never experience hot flashes; your signals may be more vague, but no less disruptive. Before you try the natural suggestions in this book or even hormone replacement therapy, you can determine your hormone levels using a simple at-home saliva test. My readers and clients have found the kit from Uni Key Health Systems especially helpful, because it includes a personalized letter of recommendations tailored to their specific test results.

Unlike the traditional blood test, the saliva test accurately measures levels of hormones that are fully active, known as bioavailable, or free, hormones. Blood hormone tests, on the other hand, measure total estrogen, which is 90 to 99 percent bound hormones. Wrapped in protein so they can be transported through the bloodstream, bound hormones are not fully biologically active. Measuring them gives you (and your doctor) a distorted picture of your hormone levels.

HOT TIMES — THE SAFE, NEW APPROACH TO TREATING MENOPAUSE

Until very recently, the medical response to the changes of menopause was to consider them symptoms of a condition that needed pharmaceutical therapy. Starting in the 1960s, estrogen replacement therapy was prescribed to replenish lost estrogen and relieve menopausal symptoms. As studies found increased rates of uterine cancer in women with intact uteruses who took ERT, progestin was added to the treatment, and hormone replacement therapy became the standard. By 2001, millions of women worldwide were taking HRT.

But all that's changed, and it couldn't have happened soon enough. Women sensed all was not well, and by mid-2002 the problems with HRT had become headline news. The Women's Health Initiative (WHI), a major U.S. study of two forms of HRT, was halted when researchers found an increased risk of heart disease, breast cancer, and blood clots in women taking Prempro. Not long after, British researchers conducting the Million Women Study reported that women who used HRT not only were more likely to develop breast cancer than women who never used HRT but also had larger tumors when diagnosed and were more likely to die from the cancer. In spring 2003, researchers in the WHI Memory Study reported that older women taking Prempro were twice as likely to develop dementia as were women taking a sugar pill (placebo). Furthermore, the risk of developing dementia doubled every five years after age 65 that a woman took HRT.

As a result of these and other findings, physicians are becoming more cautious in prescribing HRT. In an editorial accompanying the report on the WHI Memory Study in the *Journal of the American Medical Association,* the editor suggested that HRT "should not be recommended for prevention of any outcome."

Fortunately, we have more empowering choices than just taking hormone therapy or needlessly suffering through the discomforts associated with menopause. A vital and balanced diet—supplemented with vitamins, minerals, essential fatty acids, and herbs that reinforce the body's glandular system—can provide natural relief for menopausal discomforts without the known and still unknown risks inherent in hormone replacement therapy.

The Hot Times approach gives us the power to regain some control with what is going on with our bodies. Supplements, herbs, and moderation in lifestyle are all things we can use to regulate the changes that naturally occur in midlife. By making healthy choices, we can do much to minimize hot flashes and make menopause a more pleasant passage without being at the mercy of doctors and drug companies. The most common and troubling symptoms of menopause—hot flashes, sexual changes, sleep problems, weight gain, heavy bleeding, depression, irritability, and anxiety—can all be helped by the Hot Times approach.

The Hot Times Approach to Hot Flashes

Hot flashes are the most common and most distressing menopause symptom. In fact, up to 80 percent of all women experience hot flashes at some time during menopause. You may feel a sudden flush of intense heat, often beginning around your neck and face and radiating to other parts of your body. You may sweat profusely, only to get the chills a few minutes later. Your body may go into "overdrive" and your heart begin to beat rapidly. Lasting anywhere from a few minutes to a half hour, hot flashes can be accompanied by dizziness, palpitations, and heavy perspiration. If you have hot flashes during the night, they're commonly referred to as night sweats.

There are many theories as to why hot flashes occur. Some claim the estrogen/progesterone imbalance experienced at menopause sets off a reaction in the hypothalamus, which is responsible for the control of body temperature. Others say hot flashes result from increased levels of hormones secreted by the pituitary gland during menopause.

Whatever the hormonal cause, hot flashes occur when there are changes in the diameter of the blood vessels near the skin surface. These vessels dilate, allowing blood to flood into them, bringing heat to the skin surface. Although the skin temperature rises with hot flashes, the body's internal temperature does not rise and there is no fever. While hot flashes can be uncomfortable and annoying, they are not life-threatening and do go away, with or without any treatment, once the body adjusts to the changing hormone levels.

As I said, doctors have generally ignored more natural, less risky methods of relieving the discomforts of hot flashes. Sure, prescribed estrogen alleviates hot flashes by keeping blood estrogen levels artificially high. But it does not "cure" flashes, and in many cases they return once therapy is stopped. You can also take the drug clonidine, used for high blood pressure, to lessen hot flashes, but its side effects include low blood pressure, fatigue, dizziness, and headache.

More natural agents for controlling hot flashes include numerous nutrients and herbs. These substances, unlike synthetic hormones such as Premarin and Provera, don't just act to replace something that is no longer there. I believe they also provide beneficial support to the endocrine system and, in general, improve overall health.

Dietary Recommendations: Cooling Down Hot Flashes Naturally

Diet, especially as it contributes to body weight, is a key factor in controlling hot flashes. All of our lives we have been told thin is better, when in fact being a shade on the plump side is really ideal at menopause. Women who are exceptionally thin seem to suffer more during menopause, not only from hot flashes but from other estrogen-related symptoms as well, because body fat is the prime site of postmenopausal estrogen production. On the other hand, carrying around too much weight opens you up to the risk of uterine and breast cancer from the constant flow of estrogen being produced by body fat.

The use of alcohol, tobacco, and marijuana all negatively affect our hormone levels. Going "cold turkey" on these substances can do much to make our passage through menopause easier. Drinking coffee and other hot drinks, and eating hot, spicy foods and large meals appear to trigger hot flashes in some women. Substituting water or cool fruit juices for hot beverages and eating smaller meals more frequently can help.

SOY

Like many of my clients, you may find making changes in your dietary and lifestyle habits relieves hot-flash discomfort. Many women are popping soy supplements and finding creative ways to serve soy burgers, soy noodles, and the myriad other soy products introduced in recent years. Americans have been spending about $4 billion a year on soy foods, especially since 1999, when the FDA concluded that eating 25 grams of soy daily could help lower "bad" LDL cholesterol in people with high cholesterol levels. If you read the reports that the isoflavones in soy relieved hot flashes in some women, you probably thought that was a good enough reason to add soy to your diet.

In my opinion, however, the jury is still out on soy, particularly unfermented soy foods such as tofu, soy flour, soy sprouts, and soy milk. First, published reports have noted that high intake of soy foods, secondary to iodine deficiency and inadequate protein intake, creates thyroid problems. Second, while some reports have suggested the phytoestrogens in soy may protect against some forms of breast cancer, other researchers have found soy seems to encourage growth of another type of breast cancer. Finally, about one in five people is allergic to soy, causing them to experience gas, bloating, and abdominal discomfort. For clients who don't have much success with other techniques to reduce hot flashes or who want to keep soy in their diet, I recommend moderate use of the fermented soy foods tempeh and miso, along with the fermented soy supplement called Soy Essentials by Health From the Sun.

VITAMIN E

You may already be taking multiple vitamin and mineral supplements, but when you reach menopause the need for certain nutrients skyrockets. The usual one-a-day vitamin simply does not meet the requirements of your changing body. For example, the need for vitamin E increases dramatically during menopause, with some women needing ten to fifty times the usual amount.

Vitamin E has been recognized for its effectiveness against hot flashes for over fifty years. In research as far back as 1949, vitamin E was found to control severe menopausal flushing in more than 50 percent of the women studied. According to Evan Shute, a Canadian gynecologist who has been using vitamin E with his patients for the past fifty years, relief from hot flashes can be experienced after a month's use of the vitamin. It not only is helpful in regulating body temperature but is also protective of the heart (see Chapter 4), improves circulation, and helps prevent varicose veins and blood clots.

With my clients, I recommend starting off at 400 IU (international units) daily, gradually increasing the dosage in increments of 400 IU until symptoms decrease. Many women seem to find relief at levels of 1200 IU a day. A word of caution, however: if you are diabetic or taking high blood pressure medication or blood thinners, take vitamin E only under your doctor's supervision.

BIOFLAVONOIDS

In addition to vitamin E, the bioflavonoids have been found to help minimize the effects and intensity of hot flashes. These nutrients strengthen capillary walls, have a chemical activity similar to that of estrogen, and have been found to reduce the effects of hot flashes when taken regularly. One of the most popular bioflavonoids is hesperidin, the predominant flavonoid in lemons and oranges. Hesperidin seems to work by improving venous tone, restoring normal capillary permeability, and improving lymphatic drainage. It also acts on the hypothalamus, helping it to regulate temperature more easily. Hesperidin seems to work best when given along with vitamin C, so I recommend my clients take 1000 mg hesperidin and 1000 to 1500 mg vitamin C daily. Sweet oranges and tangelos are the richest dietary sources of hesperidin, along with lemons, grapes, plums, black currants, grapefruit, buckwheat, and rose hips.

ESSENTIAL FATTY ACIDS

Black currant seed oil, a balanced botanical source of the omega-3s and the essential fatty acid GLA (gamma-linolenic acid), has also been used successfully to eliminate hot flashes. Now, I know many of you might still be confused about fat. While certain fats are to be avoided, some fats are essential and must be provided in the diet because the body cannot manufacture them itself. (The topic of fat is covered in greater detail in Chapter 4.) Black currant seed oil provides a direct source of GLA, which is essential for hormone production. This essential fatty acid is also necessary for the normal functioning of the reproductive system and the adrenal glands, a source of postmenopausal hormones. In addition, essential fats are helpful in a whole host of hair, skin, and nail conditions, which will be discussed in the next section.

I've been happy to hear from a large number of menopause-age readers who followed my Two-Week Fat Flush program detailed in my best-selling book, *The Fat Flush Plan* (McGraw-Hill, 2002). *The Fat Flush Plan* features essential fats (in the form of flaxseed oil and GLA supplements), quality protein, vegetables, fruits, unsweetened cranberry juice and water, fiber, and lots of cleansing culinary herbs and spices. My readers report not only dramatic results with weight loss, but also the cessation of hot flashes and night sweats. I believe this is due to the inclusion of essential fats in the form of two tablespoonsful of high-lignan flaxseed oil, added to smoothies, salad dressings, and other no-heat recipes, as well as GLA-rich black currant seed oil taken as a supplement.

IODINE

Iodine, commonly associated with the proper functioning of your thyroid gland, is useful in reducing the occurrence of hot flashes in some women. Iodine-rich foods, eaten on a daily basis, include fish, sea vegetables, and natural iodized salt.

GAMMA-ORYZANOL

Recently, Japanese researchers have found that a substance known as gamma-oryzanol, a naturally occurring component of rice bran oil, dramatically reduces hot flashes. In amounts of 300 mg per day, gamma-oryzanol *caused an 85 percent improvement in menopausal symptoms.* Maybe the high intake of rice is the reason Japanese women don't usually suffer from hot flashes.

Herbal Remedies

Herbal remedies work well for some women, and many people are more comfortable using herbs simply because they are natural. A number of herbs have been proven effective for relieving hot flashes, including

- red clover
- ginseng
- black cohosh
- hawthorn berries
- unicorn and false unicorn root
- wild yam root
- chaste berry, or vitex
- licorice root

Red clover is available as Promensil, a supplement containing four natural plant estrogens (known as phytoestrogens or isoflavones): genistein, biochanin, diadzein, and formononetin. Studies have shown

Promensil reduces the frequency and severity of hot flashes and night sweats with no apparent side effects. Siberian ginseng, yam root, black cohosh, licorice root, and dong quai have nontoxic estrogen-like properties that act to balance hormone levels. Wild yam and vitex have progesterone-like properties. Care needs to be taken with natural licorice root, as it contains a substance that can lead to fluid and salt retention, and a few reports have been published linking black cohosh to liver damage. The unicorn roots nourish the ovaries, while the hawthorn berries contain many biologically active flavonoid compounds that are capillary-strengthening and heart-protecting.

Another popular all natural herbal remedy that has proven helpful in managing both hot flashes and mood swings is MenoCare. It contains a blend of Ayurvedic herbs such as haritaki (a rich source of vitamin C, which also acts as an adaptogen and rejuvenator), licorice, and shatavari (well known as a natural source of estrogen).

Many of these are available in tincture or capsule form at your local health food store. Follow the directions for use printed on the labels. It is very difficult to prescribe exact doses for herbal remedies, because every body responds differently. So use common sense and pay attention to your body's response.

Homeopathic Remedies

Many women are turning to the homeopathic medical system in addition to herbs. Homeopathy was founded two hundred years ago and is currently undergoing a popular renaissance here in the United States. Homeopathy uses minute dosages of natural substances to stimulate healing. One of the most common homeopathic remedies used for hot flashes is called Lachesis. This remedy, derived from the venom of a South American serpent, has proven effective in cases of severe flushing, night sweats, and headaches. The pulsatilla homeopathic formula, derived from a perennial herb known as the windflower, can be useful for more sensitive and emotional women whose hot flashes are milder in intensity. The sepia remedy, derived from the dried ink of the cuttlefish, can be used for worn-out and weakened women, while sulfur can help women who are sleepy during the day and wide awake at night. Homeopathic remedies, which are generally found in natural food stores, come in tablets formulated with milk sugar that melt under your tongue. I recommend starting with the lowest potencies; these are designated 3X, 6X, 12X, 5C, or 7C on the label (referring to the level of dilution used to make the tablet).

Many women experience relief from hot flashes with the topical use of a progesterone body cream extracted from yams grown in Mexico and converted to bioidentical progesterone in the laboratory. This natural hormone cream is absorbed through the skin and carried directly to where it is needed. Unlike the synthetic progesterones, the cream is nontoxic and without side effects because it bypasses the liver.

THE HOT TIMES APPROACH TO SEXUAL CHANGES

Increasingly, Hot Times women—women who are in midlife—who attend my lectures or visit my interactive messaging board at my website (www.annlouise.com) complain about the lack of satisfying sex in their lives and seek a remedy. Maybe you're one of them. Traditional medicine has largely ignored older women when it comes to sexual dysfunction, while offering older men Viagra and other drugs, surgical implants, and other options to ensure a long and active sex life. According to psychiatrists Barbara Bartlik and Marion Z. Goldstein, "Research on women's sexuality lags 20 years behind that for men, even though sexual dysfunction is more common in women than men."

Even if your desire is intact, you may find your sexual response and sensitivity are not what they once were, before menopause. You're less easily aroused and find yourself less sensitive to your partner's touch. Some researchers suggest age-related changes in peripheral nerves, blood vessels, and muscle tissue may play a role. Individuals with diabetes or neurologic disease may have similar nerve damage affecting their sexual response. Fatigue, from hypothyroidism or insomnia and other sleep problems, or from depression, may be contributing factors for many women. Taking steps to correct these conditions, as I describe in later sections, may be all that's needed to set your skin tingling again.

Here's some good news: celibacy is not inevitable with aging. About 70 percent of healthy 70-year-olds remain sexually active, and there are a variety of ways you can also. The first task is to pinpoint the particular reason or reasons for sexual problems you have. These reasons can include vaginal dryness that causes discomfort and lack of response; a low sex drive caused by low testosterone levels or the use of sedatives, antihistamines, or other commonly prescribed drugs; changed or decreased sexual response; and compounding health issues. As levels of estrogen decline, the vaginal walls begin to lose their elasticity and become somewhat drier and thinner. Vaginal secretions become less acidic, and there is more risk of vaginal infections. The mucous secretions from the cervix also decrease, and the vagina itself shrinks, becoming shorter and narrower. The tissues of the bladder and urethra also become more sensitive. This may increase the frequency of urination, with some women needing to void several times during the night. It can also result in increased urinary tract infections, urinary burning, and leaking of urine upon coughing, laughing, or sneezing. These changes may cause pain during intercourse and lead us to wonder whether our days of sexual pleasure are over. Luckily, many things can be done to help vaginal lubrication. Small amounts of intravaginal estriol, the safest form of estrogen, help vaginal dryness. (You can order this from a compounding pharmacy with a doctor's prescription.) There are other natural choices available, too.

Dietary Recommendations

Your lack of sensitivity during sex may be the result of vitamin or mineral imbalances, and ensuring you get enough nutrients can help restore sexual pleasure and your libido. For example, increased levels of certain minerals and vitamins—such as selenium and vitamins A, B, and C—help keep vaginal tissue membranes lubricated during and after menopause. Also, potassium stimulates the nerve center controlling contractions of the vaginal wall.

One of the best ways to find out which particular vitamins and minerals may be deficient is through a special test called a hair analysis, which measures tissue mineral levels. The hair, considered a storage organ, gives a better picture of underlying nutrient imbalances than the blood, because hair can reveal what has been going on in your body for several months. Once you've established your particular imbalances, you'll probably need to include supplements to get the levels you want. Ideally, we should get most of our vitamins and minerals from food, but modern methods of growing, harvesting, processing, and transporting food, as well as environmental stresses from tainted air and water, leave much of our food devoid of essential nutrients.

DIETARY FATS
A fat-free diet is a dangerous diet, particularly at menopause. Even some who are very nutrition-conscious and aware of health trends come to menopause with the mistaken belief that all fat is bad. What we may not be aware of, as mentioned earlier in this chapter, is that certain fats are absolutely vital to good health. You may want to refer to my book, *Supernutrition for Women* (Bantam, 2004) for complete information on the importance of the right fats to female health. In addition to their significance to hormonal regulation, essential fatty acids are crucial to the cardiovascular, immune, reproductive, and central nervous systems. More specifically, during menopause, deficiencies in these "good fats" are directly related to the drying of vagi-

nal tissue, as well as of skin, hair, and nails. Menopausal women suffering from dryness would do well to use oils like macadamia nut, olive, almond, and sesame seed for cooking and flaxseed in salad dressings or drizzled over hot veggies, because these oils provide some of the highest levels of healthy fats.

VITAMIN C

Vitamin C is particularly key to the synthesis of hormones in the adrenal glands. The adrenals, two crescent-shaped glands situated atop the kidneys, are designed to produce hormones that are converted to estrogen in body fat when ovarian hormone production slows down. (See Chapter 2 for a more extensive discussion on the role of the adrenal glands during menopause.) Animal studies have shown that the need for vitamin C increases by 75 percent during menopause, so it makes sound nutritional sense to maintain optimal levels of vitamin C—up to 5000 mg in some cases—during and after menopause. This assures that nature's backup system (the estrogen-producing mechanism of the adrenals and body fat) is adequately nourished.

VITAMINS A AND B

Vitamins A and B are essential to keeping vaginal tissues supple and responsive. The anti-infection protection from these vitamins also lessens the likelihood of vaginal infections that can interfere with sexual pleasure. Women should supplement their diets with 25,000 IU of vitamin A or the pro–vitamin A form, beta-carotene, and 50 to 100 mg of vitamin B complex daily.

VITAMIN E

Vitamin E, used both internally and topically, can be used to relieve vaginal dryness. Massaging the insides of the vagina directly with vitamin E oil can help heal dry and damaged tissue. Some women have found relief with vitamin E suppositories, used once nightly for six weeks and then once a week. Additional vitamin E through supplementation is also helpful, beginning at levels of 400 IU.

If you find that high dosages of vitamin E are not effective for you, or if you suffer from high blood pressure or take blood-thinning medication—situations where higher amounts of vitamin E are contraindicated—you may want to explore homeopathy. There are three popular homeopathic remedies women can use for vaginal dryness: lycopodium (vegetable sulfur), Natrum Muriaticum (sodium chloride), and bryonia (wild hops). Again, I suggest you start with the lower potencies or consult a trained homeopath.

ZINC

Zinc is another mineral that contributes to a healthy sexual response. Alcohol depletes your body's zinc supply, and a diet of refined white sugar and flour and other processed foods is likely to leave you with a zinc deficiency. To boost your zinc levels—and your sex life—avoid alcoholic beverages, eliminate processed foods, and add foods high in zinc, including oysters, lean red meat, pecans and most other nuts, whole eggs, and dried split peas.

POTASSIUM

If you take diuretics for high blood pressure or other conditions or, like most Americans, consume far more sodium than you need, you may be potassium-deficient. Potassium is carried out of your body in urine. To increase your potassium intake from food sources, add sea vegetables (available dried in natural food stores), sunflower seeds, almonds, and wheat germ to your diet. Avoid high-sodium foods such as olives, dill pickles, soy sauce, sauerkraut, and cheddar cheese, and, of course, take the salt shaker away from the table.

FOLIC ACID

Decreased sex drive is also one of the symptoms of a folic acid deficiency. Some experts estimate as many as 80 percent of women lack adequate folic acid. Other symptoms include moodiness, irritability, fatigue, forgetfulness, and headache—all-too-common signs of menopause as well! Try adding green leafy vegetables, tuna, salmon, cheese, brown rice, beef, beans, and barley to your diet. Alcohol depletes folic acid, so moderate your alcoholic beverage consumption.

Herbal Remedies: Who Needs Viagra?

Time and again, as I travel around the country, speak to women, and work with clients, I am asked about herbal female sexual formulas. I did some research, and I can recommend a variety of herbs that have been shown to enhance female libido, primarily by stimulating testosterone production. Try to find formulas that include at least one or more of these ingredients: damiana, ginseng, horny goat weed (also known as epimedium, or yin yang huo), saw palmetto, yohimbe, mucuna pruriens, and Tribulus terrestris.

Lifestyle: Discover These Pleasure Principles

Taking over-the-counter antihistamines and cold pills designed to dry up the nasal tissues will also dry other tissues, including those of the vagina. If you take sedatives or antidepressants, you're likely to lose your sexual desire. I urge you to talk to you doctor before you stop taking any medication, but think about what you're getting from these drugs versus what you're sacrificing. Avoid using douches and vaginal sprays, as well as colored or scented toilet paper, which can irritate sensitive vaginal tissue. Wear clothes made from natural fibers, such as cotton and silk, as they allow the skin to breathe and regulate body temperature, unlike synthetic fibers, which trap heat and moisture next to the skin.

As they say, "use it or lose it." Regular intercourse helps increase the blood flow to the vaginal tissues, which improves tone and natural lubrication. Older women who have remained sexually active throughout their lives seem to have fewer problems with vaginal dryness. Loving, relaxed foreplay can increase natural secretions, and the use of unscented lubricants like baby oil, pure aloe gel, vitamin E oil, or even borage oil during foreplay can reduce irritation and pain. Natural progesterone cream applied directly to the vagina can help dryness dramatically. A sensitive, patient lover can be a menopausal woman's best friend. Women without sexual partners can use self-stimulation to promote vaginal secretions and reduce dryness.

Certain exercises help increase vaginal blood flow, improve muscle tone, and decrease vaginal dryness. Known as the Kegel exercises, for the gynecologist who developed them, these exercises can be done anywhere at any time. To practice the Kegel exercises, simply imagine you need to stop urinating. Tighten muscles around the anus, urethra, and vagina, hold for the count of three, and then relax.

Boost Your Sex Drive and Relieve Arthritis Pain

For anyone experiencing arthritis pain, sex is likely to be the last thing on your mind. Yet it may be just what the doctor ordered! Research has found that people with arthritis can achieve up to six hours of pain relief after intercourse, probably as a result of the natural painkilling beta-endorphins released from the brain and the surge of cortisone from the adrenal glands following orgasm.

Testosterone: It's Not Just for Men

Sure it's important for vaginal health to counteract the effects of low estrogen levels. But it's equally important to boost your testosterone levels if you want to keep the fires of sexual desire burning into menopause and beyond. One way to restore your testosterone levels is to use natural progesterone, the precursor to testosterone. Many women experience not only a boost in their sex drive but also improved mood, decreased anxiety, enhanced sleep, and increased energy when they use progesterone. Some alternative medicine professionals go even further in their support of progesterone—they believe it stimulates new bone formation, protecting against osteoporosis, although the USFDA-approved study of progesterone cream found no statistically significant increase in bone density over placebo.

The easiest way to use progesterone is in a transdermal cream with 400 to 600 mg progesterone per ounce. You simply rub ¼ to ½ teaspoon twice daily (for a dose of 20 to 30 mg) onto an area with relatively thin skin, such as your face, neck around the thyroid, inner arm, or palm of your hand. The progesterone is quickly absorbed into the underlying fat layer, where the capillaries pick it up for movement into your bloodstream. An added benefit of the cream is the moisturizing effect many women experience from the cream on dry skin.

Progesterone is also available in a vitamin E oil that you take three to four times a day by putting a few drops of it under your tongue and holding it there for about a minute. You can take natural progesterone capsules, but because 85 to 90 percent will be excreted through the liver, you will need to take 100 to 200 mg a day to get the effect of the cream form.

THE HOT TIMES APPROACH TO SLEEP PROBLEMS

Women are probably the most sleep-deprived creatures on earth. At least that's what Joyce A. Walsleben, director of the Sleep Disorders Center at the New York University School of Medicine, suggests. Many menopausal women would agree with her. Some of the reasons older women can't get to sleep or wake often during the night are the same as those of younger women—stress, anxiety, or pain, for example. Even if you've slept like a baby all your life, menopause and its hormonal fluctuations may cause sleep problems for the first time in your life. Night sweats, those nocturnal hot flashes that wake many women lying in perspiration-soaked sheets, often leave sufferers unable to get back to sleep. Following my suggestions outlined earlier to relieve hot flashes may eliminate night sweats as well.

A Hidden Cause of Sleep Disturbances

One largely overlooked cause of sleep disturbances is an infestation of parasites. Unless they've traveled aboard recently, few Americans suspect a roundworm or amoeba of causing their night sweats, insomnia, or wakefulness. Yet experts estimate at least 50 percent of adult Americans may be carrying a parasite, which releases toxic substances and sets off a chronic immune challenge, including surges in cortisol. If your sleep problems persist after you've tried other Hot Times suggestions, you may want to cleanse your system using Uni Key's Para and/or Verma Systems. I have used these in my practice for years for unresolved symptoms of all kinds. My book *Guess What Came to Dinner?: Parasites and Your Health* (Avery) tells the whole story.

Insomnia and Obesity: Don't Let Your Sleeping Habits Weigh You Down

Who knew? Insomnia can make you fat! A study published in 2000 by the University of Chicago's Department of Medicine revealed that too little sleep impairs the way your body handles food, creating impaired glucose tolerance. This can result in insulin resistance and obesity. A lack of quality sleep, known as deep, or rapid-eye-movement (REM), sleep, probably impedes surges of growth hormone, resulting in increased fat tissue and reduced muscle mass. Sleep deprivation also causes lower body temperature and fatigue, which usually lead to increased food consumption as your body seeks to boost energy and help you stay warm. Additional research has led the Chicago scientists to conclude that chronic sleep deprivation can also contribute to both the onset and severity of diabetes and high blood pressure.

Sleep and the adrenal hormone cortisol are entwined. Insufficient sleep forces your cortisol levels to rise and stay elevated. Research has shown that someone 50 years old may have evening cortisol levels as much as thirty times higher than a younger person. Chronically high cortisol levels disturb moods and even sleep, as well as contributing to weight gain. Cortisol works in concert with other chemicals to quicken fat storage, targeting the central fat cells. It releases glucose and fatty acids so that muscles have energy, stimulating your appetite to encourage you to replenish fuel. Consequently, when you can't sleep, your cortisol levels rise and suddenly you find yourself wanting to grab a late-night eclair, which only aggravates the situation by promoting even more cortisol production.

I've devoted an entire chapter (Chapter 2) to the proper functioning and nurturing of those powerhouses, the adrenal glands. Follow my suggestions to ensure adrenal health and you may find your sleep problems disappear as your cortisol levels stabilize.

Dietary Recommendations: Eat Your Way to a Better Night's Sleep

Mineral imbalances often lead to insomnia. One of these involves the interrelationship between copper and zinc. The levels of these minerals tend to work in opposition; that is, when serum copper levels are high, zinc levels are low. The ideal ratio seems to be one part copper to eight parts zinc. Both minerals are essential to almost every function in our bodies. Among other activities, copper stimulates production of neurotransmitters such as epinephrine and dopamine, which heightens brain and nervous system activity. Brain stimulation is the last thing you need when you're trying to go to sleep!

If you are still consuming the typical low-fat, high-carbohydrate diet, you may have a zinc deficiency accompanied by copper overload. The carbohydrates in these diets are usually highly processed breads, pastas, muffins, and bagels. Any zinc contained in the grains was removed in milling. These diets are also low in fiber, needed to aid copper detoxification. Finally, eating less animal protein means you're getting less zinc from these important food sources. Protein is also needed for the liver to use and transport copper properly. Factors that often contribute to a zinc deficiency, an excess of copper, or both are taking medications such as diuretics, cortisone, and antacids; consuming alcoholic beverages and coffee; living with significant stress; and experiencing illness or surgery.

Mineral imbalances can be corrected with a combination of diet and supplements. Avoid high-copper foods such as oysters, liver, brewer's yeast, tea made from tea bags, and cocoa powder. Include lean meat, poultry, and eggs to boost your zinc intake, and consider taking 15 to 50 mg zinc supplement daily. If you feel you are overconsuming copper in foods, look for copper-free supplements. With this requirement in mind, I formulated a copper-free, hypoallergenic multiple vitamin, mineral, and plant enzyme complex product called the Uni Key Female Multiple.

Another commonly deficient mineral can lead to sleepless nights: Too little magnesium can cause you to wake up repeatedly during the night. It's also a factor in muscle cramps and spasms that can interrupt sleep, primarily because of an excess of calcium (see Chapter 3). Among the factors depleting your magnesium stores are consuming coffee, sugar, colas, and alcoholic beverages and taking diuretics. Diabetes, hypothyroidism, and chronic pain can also affect your levels of magnesium, as can a diet high in sodium, calcium, or carbohydrates.

At the same time, moderate your calcium consumption. (I know this flies in the face of current advice; see page 67 for more information about the effects of too much calcium.) Add high-magnesium foods such as nuts, dried apricots and figs, whole-wheat bread, sea vegetables, spinach, and most dried beans. Once your magnesium levels have stabilized, if you want to take a calcium supplement, look for one with an equal part magnesium, such as OsteoKey (available from Uni Key Health Systems), which includes 800 mg calcium (in the highly bioavailable form hydroxyapatite) and 800 mg magnesium (carbonate and aspartate forms). The Female Multiple can also help you get your calcium-magnesium ratio in balance, with the supplement's 2:1 formula of magnesium to calcium. You can also find straight magnesium supplements at most health food stores. Start at 400 mg daily and gradually work your way up to tolerance levels. Magnesium has the added benefit of acting as a natural laxative.

Supplements and Herbal Remedies:
Some Relaxing Tips

You may find several other supplements have a calming effect that promotes sleep. GABA, or gamma-aminobutyric acid, is an inhibitory neurotransmitter made in the brain from the amino acid glutamate with the aid of vitamin B_6. GABA encourages relaxation, analgesia, and sleep by inhibiting nerve impulses and preventing stress-related messages from reaching the brain. Supplement your brain's production by taking 500 to 750 mg twice a day.

The herb valerian is well known for its sedative qualities and its ability to relax the central nervous system and the smooth-muscle groups. It has been used as a sleeping aid for hundreds of years, especially by people who are excited or have difficulty in falling to sleep because of nervousness. The recommended dose is 600 mg taken two hours before bedtime; it may take up to four weeks to produce results.

Lifestyle

Don't overlook the value of exercise to induce sleep. A 2003 Seattle study of women age 50 to 75 who were not taking HRT and were having sleep problems found that the women who exercised aerobically (walking or biking) in the mornings for 3.5 to 4 hours per week had significantly less trouble falling asleep. Even women who simply carried out low-intensity stretching exercises for several hours a week saw some improvement. Just avoid performing vigorous exercise in the evening, if sleep eludes you. You'll find my Hot Times Exercise Prescription described in Chapter 6.

THE HOT TIMES APPROACH TO HEAVY BLEEDING

Heavy and irregular bleeding are among the most common symptoms of menopause and make life miserable for those of us experiencing them. While usually resulting from fluctuating hormone levels and the production of too much estrogen and not enough progesterone, heavy and irregular bleeding can be caused by many other factors, including stress, smoking, alcohol, spicy foods, and caffeine. Fibroid tumors in the uterus can also cause heavy bleeding. The good news is that fibroids are usually benign, and in most women do not require surgery, as they will shrink during menopause because of decreased estrogen production. However, uterine and cervical cancer can also cause heavy bleeding, so these conditions need to be ruled out. Yearly Pap smears can detect any negative changes in cervical tissue and should be a part of every woman's routine health checkups, even past menopause. A pelvic ultrasound probe called vaginal sonography can uncover fibroid tumors, cysts, thickening of the endometrium, and uterine cancer.

Dietary Recommendations:
Find a Careful Iron Balance

In all cases of excessive blood loss, iron-deficiency anemia can result. To avoid this, include good sources of dietary iron like red meat, dark green leafy vegetables, beans, and beets in your diet. Supplementing with vitamin C or eating vitamin C–rich foods may be helpful, as vitamin C aids in iron absorption. Increasing the intake of specific iron-rich foods, with accompanying vitamin C, works well for some women. Those who have had chronic anemia may require more concentrated measures. Supplementation with liquid iron preparations, which are less likely than iron pills to cause constipation, should be considered.

On the other hand, if you are not anemic, iron supplementation may be unwise. It is important to note that research suggests that excess stored iron may be a factor in both heart disease and cancer. Unlike most other minerals, excess iron is not eliminated through the kidneys. It accumulates and generates free radicals. Among other destructive activities, these free radicals lead to oxidation of cholesterol, associated with heart disease. If you are no longer losing iron monthly via menstruation, iron overload can become a problem. You may want to request that your nutritionally oriented physician run both a hemoglobin anemia and serum ferritin test. The serum ferritin test is the best way to find out if you are storing excess iron in the body.

Homeopathic Remedies

Homeopathic practitioners have found several remedies stop excessive menstrual bleeding, including homeopathic phosphorus and homeopathic belladonna. Consult a practitioner for a tincture to be created specifically for your symptoms, or look for products at your local health food store. Follow the package label directions, and select the lowest potencies first (3X, 6X, 12X, 5C, or 7C). Once you find relief, you can taper your dosage to the lowest level that still keeps symptoms from reappearing.

Lifestyle

If you suffer from heavy bleeding, take a close look at your lifestyle. Excessive use of alcohol and frequent use of aspirin both negatively affect the blood's ability to clot and lead to increased blood flow. Couch potatoes, beware—lack of exercise can also contribute to heavy menstrual bleeding. Consistent, strenuous exercise lowers estrogen production in the ovaries by inhibiting the production of pituitary hormones. Avoid those long soaks in a hot bath or shower during periods of heavy bleeding, because heat dilates blood vessels, thereby increasing blood flow.

THE HOT TIMES APPROACH TO DEPRESSION, IRRITABILITY, AND ANXIETY

No, you're not crazy, nor is it all in your head. It's true that many women experience mood swings, anxiety, insomnia (sometimes related to hot flashes and night sweats), and depression during the menopausal years. But no psychological disorder has ever been attributed directly to menopause. These psychological symptoms can and do occur in women throughout their lives. Unfortunately, in our culture, many women's emotional responses and/or reactions are often blamed on hormones—it's either "that time of the month" or "that time of life." But studies show that when compared with younger women, women in the menopausal age group show a significant drop in psychological symptoms. This is not to say that fluctuating hormone levels don't leave many of us experiencing correspondingly fluctuating mood swings during this time. These hormone-related mood swings, like those associated with PMS, can throw us for a loop. During menopause, depression and mood swings can be related to the imbalance of estrogen and progesterone. It is important to remember that although uncomfortable and sometimes frightening, mood swings are not long-term and do go away as the body adjusts to your lowered estrogen levels.

Shifting moods and feelings of depression during menopause may result from social and environmental stresses in combination with hormonal changes. Because women in menopause don't share a pattern of symptoms, many of us really don't know what to expect during this time and describe feeling anxious and out of control. Lack of information about the physical changes we are experiencing can contribute to the intensity of these feelings.

Midlife entails many more life changes than just menopause. Our children leave home and our focus on child-rearing ends, and unless women have developed their own interests or careers, this change can lead to feelings of personal emptiness. Some women mourn the loss of their ability to bear more children. Also, your own parents may have reached an age when they need to be cared for. And some become single for the first time in many years, through divorce or death. Depression is an understandable reaction to the many external changes that may be taking place at this time of life.

Prescribing tranquilizers or antidepressants for menopausal women with anxiety or depression has been common medical practice for many years, one that does little to identify or solve the root of the problem. Furthermore, it introduces addictive substances with unpleasant side effects into a body that is already out of biochemical balance, thereby increasing the potential for further physical and psychological problems.

Supplements and Herbal Remedies: Balance Your Mood

Fluctuating estrogen levels affect both calcium and magnesium metabolism, two minerals important for the nourishment and health of the nervous system, as well as of bones and the heart (as we will explore in later chapters). Maintaining a healthy calcium/magnesium balance is vital, yet so many menopausal women take calcium supplements with no regard for this important biochemical balance. A high intake of calcium without accompanying magnesium can increase magnesium requirements and intensify magnesium-deficiency symptoms, such as nervousness, anxiety, and depression. My research suggests that menopausal women should take one part calcium to one part magnesium.

Stress-fighting B vitamins and amino acids can do much to decrease anxiety and depression and improve our sense of well-being. In particular, inositol has been found to lessen anxiety. Foods such as wheat germ, whole-wheat bread, oatmeal, and various dried beans are good dietary sources of inositol. If you take a vitamin B complex supplement, look for one with at least 100 mg inositol. At the same time, be sure to eliminate vitamin robbers like caffeine, alcohol, sugar, aluminum, soda pop, and certain medications like antacids, antibiotics, and diuretics.

Several herbs exert a natural calming effect, relieving anxiety and promoting sleep. These include Saint-John's-wort, kava, passionflower, skullcap, camomile, and valerian root. They can be taken in capsule form or as alcohol-free tinctures or made into teas. Be sure to follow the directions on the label.

Lifestyle: Relax!

If you haven't found time for rest and relaxation before this point in your life—and too many of us haven't—midlife anxiety and depression may give you new reasons to start taking more time for yourself. Taking time out of every day to exercise, relax, meet friends, seek counseling, or join a menopause support or discussion group will not only help you cope with your menopause symptoms but also allow you to work more effectively at your job and family responsibilities.

Brisk walking, biking, jumping on a mini-trampoline, and other forms of cardiovascular exercise increase oxygen flow to your brain, which will give you more energy and less anxiety. Regular exercise also stimulates production of your body's "happy hormones," endorphins, which elevate mood and help you feel in control. The Hot Times Exercise Prescription, described in Chapter 6, is a daily program with cardiovascular, muscle-strengthening, and flexibility exercises. Give yourself thirty minutes to an hour a day and see how great you can feel.

Relaxation techniques are highly individual—what calms one person has no effect on another. So experiment. Among the techniques you might want to try are aromatherapy with a daily twenty-minute soak in a hot bath fragrant with rose or lavender essential oil, a weekly massage to release those endorphins and boost oxygen flow, or daily meditation. You could also release tension by stimulating your creative right brain with a painting class or with writing in a journal.

Reach out to others. Call a friend, do lunch, or sign up for volunteer work. Join a menopause discussion/support group through your local women's health center or find one online (see Resources). If your depression or anxiety seems overwhelming, try professional counseling.

THE HOT TIMES APPROACH
TO WEIGHT GAIN

The preliminary results of a survey conducted by Judith Wurtman of the Massachusetts Institute of Technology indicate that 65 to 75 percent of women involuntarily gain weight at menopause. This weight gain was experienced by women going through both natural and surgically induced menopause, and it appears that a slightly higher percentage of women on hormone therapy gained weight compared with those women who took no hormones. Interestingly, these percentages coincide with the percentage of women who experience symptomatic difficulties during menopause.

Those extra pounds that show up at menopause may be due to a lack of progesterone and the consequent estrogen dominance. This is something farmers have known for years, which is why the synthetic estrogen hormone diethylstilbesterol (DES) is given to steers to fatten them up. Another reason for menopausal weight gain relates to the decline in ovulation. During the first ten days to two weeks of our menstrual cycle, our bodies use up a substantial number of calories in the process of ovulation. So when we stop ovulating (enter menopause), we are left with extra calories, up to 300 daily in some cases, that are not being burned. Unfortunately, many of these excess calories will end up where we least want to see them if we don't compensate by decreasing our caloric intake or increasing our physical activity. Weight gain during and after menopause may also result from negative attitudes about aging and perceived loss of sexual attractiveness, as many of us choose to compensate for this perceived loss through food, and a lot of the foods that we turn to for comfort— creamy, rich, and sweet—are heavy in nutritionally empty calories.

Dietary Recommendations

As discussed earlier, poor dietary habits throughout a lifetime come home to roost during the Hot Times transition. What you could get away with in your 20s and 30s is quite a different dietary story in your 40s and 50s, without the balancing ability of a more youthful metabolism. Changing your diet can at times seem overwhelming. A lifetime of eating habits will not be unlearned overnight. You will do well to make your dietary changes one step at a time. A good way to start is by keeping a three-day food journal. This can help to reveal if you are overdoing unhealthy foods (such as fried foods, sugars, and refined, chemicalized, and processed foods) and not including enough nutritious foods (like fresh fruits, vegetables, whole grains, and proteins from fish, poultry, eggs, and beans).

It is important to limit nonessential fats, which are saturated fats found in pork and full-fat dairy products like cheese and ice cream. Hydrogenated fats, found in margarines and vegetable shortenings, function like saturated fats in the body and also inhibit essential fatty acid metabolism, so hydrogenated fats should be avoided as well. Your diet should consist of vegetables, fruits, legumes, whole grains, and quality protein. The Hot Times Diet, Chapter 7, and the menus and recipes in Chapter 8 will help to simplify these changes. This diet plan will help you not only lose weight but also avoid many of the other midlife health problems, such as osteoporosis and heart disease. It's always been important to eat a healthy, balanced diet, but your body needs it even more now as it goes through additional hormonal changes.

How fortunate we are to be living in the twenty-first century, when we can choose from a full range of options, both conventional and alternative, to treat our most prevalent symptoms. With time, your night sweats, sleep disturbances, moodiness, and weight gain may all be a thing of the past as you discover the best natural remedy for your changing body.

TWO

Get Rid of Stress: Discover the Secrets to a Worry-Free Menopause

I DON'T NEED TO TELL YOU THAT WOMEN ARE UNDER A GREAT deal of stress. As you read this, your cell phone will probably ring, your in-box will fill with e-mail messages, or your partner or children will come looking to you for help. You may even be responsible for caring for your aging parents. Stress isn't new, of course, and our bodies have complex systems to help us cope with physical, emotional, and mental stress. But those systems, as good as they are, are not invincible. Add the physical changes of menopause to other common midlife stresses and you're set up for system collapse.

THE STRESS OF MENOPAUSE: AN OVERTAXED ADRENAL SYSTEM

When we enter menopause, nature doesn't simply turn off our hormones and expect us to compensate with synthetic hormone replacement therapy. A natural backup system, consisting of the adrenal glands and our own body fat, is designed to make up for the declining hormone output. However, the years of enduring the stresses of modern-day living severely compromise the ability of this secondary system to function.

After menopause, the ovaries continue to produce some estrogen at a lower, more consistent level, as well as androgens, hormones similar to male hormones. Androgens play an important role in sexuality and health and promote muscle strength, vaginal elasticity, and sex drive. Research has shown that even women in their eighties continue to produce small amounts of androgens. Androgens are converted to estrogen in your body fat, but the ovaries are not the primary source of these important hormones.

The adrenal glands produce 80 percent of the androgens circulating in our bodies, and they are used by our bodies' fat stores to produce estrogen. In essence, our body fat functions like another gland, producing estrogen from raw materials (androgens) and storing it for future release. The amount of estrogen converted in the body's fat is directly related to the amount of body fat present. This is why very thin women (those with less than 18 percent body fat) seem to have more symptoms associated with their menopause. Being overweight isn't the answer either, however, as overweight women (those who are more than 25 percent above the ideal weight for their height) have a higher risk of breast and uterine cancer, because their body fat is constantly storing and releasing high levels of estrogen for long periods of time.

Androgen-based estrogen protects women from uncomfortable menopausal body changes, but only about 25 percent of us seem to produce enough of this type of estrogen to be able to sail through menopause comfortably. The other 75 percent may suffer from adrenal insufficiency, exhaustion, or hypoadrenia, a condition in which the adrenals are not capable of meeting all the demands placed upon them.

Androgens are by no means the only hormones produced by the two small glands nestled atop the kidneys. The adrenal cortex, the outer portion of the glands, produces more than thirty different steroids and hormones, including aldosterone and cortisol. Aldosterone helps control the flow of sodium and potassium in and out of cells. Cortisol plays multiple roles in some of the common signs of menopause.

In addition to the emotional and mental stress we commonly think of, physical stress—including injury, overwork, and lack of sleep—puts stress on our body, specifically the adrenal glands. The adrenals regulate hormone production and the processing of any chemical substance, whether from environmental pollutants or diets high in refined and overprocessed foods, that must be detoxified by our bodies. This, too, puts stress on the glands and can eventually lead to adrenal burnout. In addition, job pressures; lack of or excessive exercise; use of stimulants such as coffee, sugar, and "recreational" drugs; and tumultuous personal relationships can contribute to adrenal burnout. Our bodies react in the same manner no matter what produces the stress. Those of us who live with constant, unending worries about finances, children, health problems (either our own or those of someone we love), divorce, and other concerns use up excessive amounts of nutritional reserves every day, which only adds to the body's overload. And chances are, if we're "stressed out," we're not eating well to begin with.

Your Body's Reaction to Stress

Hans Selye, M.D., a pioneer in the area of stress research and the adrenal glands, recognized that stress, no matter what the source, will cause the body to use vitamins and minerals in great amounts, beyond its normal needs. Dr. Selye described what is known as the general adaption syndrome (GAS), noting that stress triggers three distinct stages or reactions:

- **Stage 1: The Alarm Reaction.** In the alarm reaction, the body prepares for stress. The adrenals begin to "hyperfunction," producing extra amounts of hormones to respond to the stress alarm. This is one of the normal functions for which the adrenals were designed. Once the stress is removed, the adrenals quiet down and return to their normal functioning.

- **Stage 2: The Resistance Stage.** If the stress continues for a long period, the body enters the resistance stage. The adrenals begin to adapt by actually increasing their size and function. In order to do this, however, energy is drawn from the body's reserves. Nutrients not supplied by the diet are siphoned off from reserve areas. This resistance stage can continue for weeks, months, and even years, until the body weakens from lack of reserves of both energy and nutrition.
- **Stage 3: The Exhaustion Stage.** In the exhaustion stage, the body's reserves of both energy and nutrition are exhausted. The body can take only so much abuse. The antistress mechanisms are gone and there is nothing left in reserve. This stage of exhaustion, often expressed as fatigue or chronic tiredness, is one of the most common complaints in our culture.

As you can well imagine, by the time many of us enter menopause, our adrenal glands are either in a state of constant hyperfunction or in burnout. Hyperfunctioning adrenals can result in many of the same symptoms attributed to menopause itself—high blood pressure, dizziness, headaches, hot flashes, excessive facial and body hair growth, and other masculine tendencies. Adrenal burnout can also lead to allergies, low blood sugar, and diabetes, which will be discussed in Chapter 5. The chronic mental and emotional stress we live with, combined with poor dietary and lifestyle habits, severely compromises these tiny glands. Not only do they no longer function adequately in response to stress, they are incapable of producing those beneficial androgens that could alleviate many of our menopausal discomforts.

The Cortisol Connection

Cortisol is one of several hormones secreted to provide energy in response to stress. Cortisol stimulates the release of protein from muscle so it can be converted to glucose, inhibits protein synthesis, increases the release of fatty acids from fat tissue, and stimulates the conversion of noncarbohydrates to glucose. All of the resulting extra blood sugar provides the fuel you need to respond to an immediate stress.

But what happens if stress continues indefinitely, as is the case for so many of us juggling careers, family, and menopausal changes? Then cortisol levels remain high, as do glucose levels. According to the research conducted by Pamela Peeke, M.D., at the National Institutes of Health, if this excess blood sugar is not used for energy production, it is stored as fat, usually in your abdominal area. Central fat cells are deep abdominal visceral cells that have four times more cortisol receptors than the fat cells found just beneath the skin. Consequently, cortisol is drawn to the central fat cells, where it activates enzymes to store fat. This process is what gives you that midlife tummy bulge that's so difficult to lose.

Cortisol influences overall weight gain in other ways as well. Increased levels of the hormone set off food cravings, especially for high-fat, high-carbohydrate foods, leading you to take in many more calories than you need. Cortisol also brings about the breakdown of muscle tissue, which causes your metabolism to drop and makes it harder for you to lose weight or to maintain weight loss.

Cortisol affects the way you sleep, too. Under healthy circumstances, cortisol levels are highest in the morning to give you the energy you need to face the day. Then by evening, levels fall by about 90 percent, allowing you to get a full night's sleep. At least one study has found that women with family responsibilities and jobs tend to have elevated cortisol levels at night. Other studies have found evening cortisol levels rise as we age. Both of these factors may help account for the fragmented sleep and lack of deep, or rapid-eye-movement (REM), sleep many menopausal women experience.

Cortisol's effects on weight gain can also be partly explained by its connection to the functioning of the thyroid gland. One of the ingredients needed to make cortisol is the amino acid tyrosine, which is also required by the thyroid gland to make thyroid hormone. As supplies of tyrosine are consumed to make excess cortisol, levels of thyroid hormone decline. This results in fatigue, weight gain, and hypothyroidism. This condition is so common in menopausal women that I've devoted an entire section to it in Chapter 5. Producing cortisol also uses another ingredient, dehydroepiandrosterone (DHEA), needed to produce sex hormones. As DHEA levels decline, so do those of the sex hormones, leading to a lower sex drive.

Excess cortisol is associated with a wide range of other effects, including

- increased cholesterol and triglyceride levels
- increased blood pressure
- increased insulin levels
- short-term memory loss
- damage to nerve and brain tissue
- decreased regeneration of connective tissue, related to wound healing and bone health
- decreased serotonin, leading to irritability, depression, and anxiety

Knowing When You're Too Stressed: Understanding Adrenal Burnout

Early-warning signs of adrenal insufficiency include chronic low blood pressure, fatigue, low stamina, sensitivity to cold, and addictions to either sweet or salty foods. Women who consider themselves "night people" often suffer from adrenal exhaustion or burnout. These women are usually tired when they get up and spend the better part of the day spiking their tired adrenal glands with caffeine, nicotine, sugar, sodas, or excessive exercise. At the end of the day, their burned-out but artificially stimulated adrenals are giving them energy to go all night. This cycle is a red flag for adrenal problems in women.

The simplest and best test to identify hidden adrenal burnout is known as the postural blood pressure test. It is a good idea to have your doctor do this test for you routinely so that you can detect the problem before it is full-blown. To take the test, you will be placed in a reclining position for four or five minutes and your doctor will record your blood pressure. You will then be asked to move to a standing position and the doctor will take a second blood pressure reading. The difference in blood pressure levels is the key to diagnosing hypo-functioning adrenal glands. In a body with healthy glands, blood pressure will show only an insignificant drop, if any at all. But when the difference in the two blood pressures is severe, hypoadrenalism is strongly indicated. Blood pressure in individuals with this condition has been known to drop as much as forty points.

THE HOT TIMES APPROACH TO DESTRESSING THROUGH ADRENAL SUPPORT

When stress hits, our nutritional needs skyrocket and remain higher than normal as long as the stress remains. Whether the stress you feel comes from mental or physical sources, or from the physical and emotional changes of menopause, nutrition is the key to protecting your body from its damaging effects. We need to fortify our bodies with nutrients from both diet and supplements every day so that our reserves are not depleted in times of stress. Adequate protein—as well as a number of vitamins, minerals, and herbs—can support and enhance adrenal function during this time.

Dietary Recommendations

Stress can deplete the stores of the minerals magnesium, calcium, zinc, potassium, sodium, and copper from your body's tissues. Unfortunately, dietary deficiencies in these important minerals are already common because of soil exhaustion, overprocessing of foods, careless cooking habits, and the eating of nutritionally empty junk foods.

To support your adrenal system, be sure to include mineral-rich foods in your diet. Minerally packed foods include all of the richly colored fruits and vegetables: green vegetables, such as broccoli, collards, kale, and mustard greens; the yellow-orange vegetables, such as squash, pumpkin, carrots, and sweet potatoes; and fruits, such as bananas, strawberries, and cantaloupe. Legumes have a high iron content, and fermented soy products like miso and tempeh are rich in copper. Sources of manganese include leafy greens, sea vegetables, whole-grain cereals, nuts, and seeds. Lean red meats, eggs, seafood, pumpkin seeds, and whole grains supply ample amounts of zinc, and are important especially for women.

The very best food sources of naturally balanced minerals come from the sea. Sea vegetables, sold in dried form in health food stores, provide high amounts of magnesium, potassium, phosphorus, iodine, iron, and other key trace minerals like manganese, chromium, selenium, and zinc. You may not be familiar with sea vegetables, but they should be present in every woman's pantry because of their extraordinary nutrient content. They are also versatile and can be used as side dishes and condiments.

Hijiki, for example, a sea vegetable that tastes a bit like licorice and looks like tangled black strings, contains significant amounts of both iron and calcium. One-half cup of cooked hijiki is higher in iron content than two eggs and contains almost the same amount of calcium as one-half cup of milk. Sea vegetables are also high in protein. Nori, a nutty-tasting seaweed that comes in sheets and is used with sushi, contains almost 30 percent protein. It can be toasted and crumbled over fish, vegetables, and pasta. I recommend that my clients toast a sheet of nori every morning and crumble it over their whole-grain cereal. In addition to being a good source of minerals, sea vegetables like blue-green algae or spirulina, kelp, nori, arame, wakame, hijiki, and sea palms contain a substance called sodium alginate that pulls toxic heavy metals from the system. My Spring Minestrone (see page 216) is another tasty way to enjoy these nutrient-rich vegetables.

The B-complex vitamins, known as the antistress vitamins, are crucial during stress. Even a slight lack of vitamin B_2 can cause adrenal gland damage. Pantothenic acid is essential to the production of many of the adrenal hormones; it also nourishes the adrenals, and a deficiency of this important B vitamin can cause atrophy of the glands. The best dietary sources of B-complex vitamins are desiccated liver, legumes, blackstrap molasses, and whole grains.

The need for vitamin C has been found to increase dramatically during times of stress, with our bodies needing as much as two and a half times more than normal. Vitamin C–rich fruits and vegetables include citrus fruits, cantaloupe, green peppers, and broccoli.

A surprising number of my clients suffering from adrenal burnout report strong cravings for chocolate. Interestingly, chocolate is a fairly high source of both magnesium and copper, two of the essential minerals required for energy production in the adrenals. Chocolate's call may indeed be the body crying for nutrients that have been lost because of stress. Obviously, chocolate is a poor choice for magnesium and copper supplementation because it contains large amounts of sugar and saturated fats. When you feel this craving, instead of having some chocolate, try to include more mineral-rich foods in your next meal.

To ensure that the foods you buy don't lose their vitamin and mineral content during shipping, try to purchase foods that are locally grown. Labels that certify that the produce is organically grown provide good assurance that no pesticides or herbicides have been used in the growing process.

Supplements and Herbal Remedies

I always recommend the Uni Key Adrenal Formula (see Resources) to my clients with symptoms of adrenal burnout. The caplets contain vitamins A, B_5, B_6, and C, zinc, tyrosine, and freeze-dried raw bovine adrenal, adrenal cortex, spleen, and liver tissue concentrates. I have taken this supplement myself for over ten years. If you're experiencing high stress or long-term chronic stress, include up to 3000 mg of vitamin C, taken in small doses throughout the day for optimum absorption.

Herbs can also come to the rescue to help reduce stress, alleviating the strain on the adrenals. Hops, passionflower, skullcap, and Chinese or American ginseng are all beneficial. Numerous studies have shown that ginseng is an adaptogen, which means it helps the body adapt to excessive stressful states. Hops, passionflower, and skullcap all have the ability to act as natural sedatives, calming the nervous system and relieving headaches and insomnia. These herbs are all available in capsule form, and as nonalcoholic tinctures and herbal teas. A good herbal source of vitamin C is rose hip tea.

The best herbal strategy for combating stress is to put a blend of herbs to work. The formula StressCare contains several herbs, including Ashwagandha and Chyavanprash, which are blended to work synergistically to calm tension and rejuvenate your body. Ashwagandha supports the adrenal glands by delivering restorative micronutrients. Chyavanprash contains forty different ingredients and is rich in antioxidants, especially bioflavonoids that support the absorption of vitamin C. StressCare, which also contains the effective nerve tonic mucuna, has been found effective against stress-related conditions like premature aging, fatigue, insomnia, and emotional imbalance. You can find this supplement at health food stores and on www.himalayausa.com.

Gamma-aminobutyric acid (GABA), an inhibitory neurotransmitter made in the brain from the amino acid glutamate and vitamin B_6, prevents stress overload on your adrenals. It is known to encourage relaxation, analgesia, and sleep by inhibiting nerve impulses and preventing stress-related messages from reaching the brain. Supplement your brain's production by taking 500 to 750 mg twice a day.

Lifestyle

You can help your adrenal glands recover from exhaustion and lessen the stress in your life by trying some or all of the following suggestions:

- Simplify your life. When adrenal burnout hits, your energy is needed for healing. Cut back on social activities and obligations that create stress and rob you of energy.
- Take some time every day for relaxation, recreation, and exercise. Initially you may find you have little energy for exercise, so start slow and build up. Be gentle with yourself. (See Chapter 6 for exercise recommendations.)
- Learn to take control of your life and your time. Once we accept responsibility for our lives and stop blaming other people and circumstances, we can begin to use our energy to solve problems.
- Break the worry habit. The energy wasted worrying can be used in your healing process.
- Learn to share your feelings, both negative and positive. Join a support group. Learning to release pent-up angers and frustrations can help lessen your emotional burdens.
- Find something safe to hit—punch a pillow or hit a tennis ball—to release pent-up emotions.
- Develop good sleeping habits and make sure your body gets adequate rest.

As you can see, the real secret to a stress-free, worry-free menopause lies in the glands—the adrenal glands, to be exact. In the case of the adrenals, many of us would feel better if we knew better. Because we have been completely unaware of their existence—let alone their function—we have abused and neglected them through diet and bad lifestyle habits, such as ingesting too much coffee, alcohol, and sugar. But now you know how vital these tiny glands are for backup hormone support during and after menopause. Nurture and regenerate these "forgotten" glands and they can supply your body with adequate levels of hormones to help ease your transition through menopause.

THREE

Osteoporosis: Much More Than a Deficiency Disease

WHEN WE WERE KIDS, A BROKEN BONE MAY HAVE KEPT US off the volleyball court or lost us the lead in the school play. We were devastated at the time, but we quickly recovered. Not so at midlife and beyond. For those of us who develop osteoporosis, a hip fracture can be fatal. But it doesn't have to be. Once we understand how our bone structure works and what the latest research findings tell us, we can put the Hot Times approach into action to stay straight and strong. Whether you are at high risk for osteoporosis or are already in the early or late stages of this disease, read on—the recommendations in this chapter are just what the nutritionist ordered.

WHY OSTEOPOROSIS MATTERS

- About 8 million American women suffer from osteoporosis, and three times that number are at risk.
- One in two women over age 50 will break a bone in her lifetime.

- More women die each year from osteoporosis-related injuries than die from ovarian and breast cancer combined.
- 1.5 million osteoporosis-related fractures happen in the United States annually.
- Direct health care costs related to these fractures exceeds $47 million a day.

We now know osteoporosis is not simply a "calcium-deficiency disease" or even a "hormone-deficiency disease" that can be cured by taking calcium supplements or hormone replacement therapy. It is a complex condition that develops slowly over a period of years before it reaches the stage where it can be diagnosed. Historically, diagnosis usually came as a result of fractures, when brittleness was already substantially established. Standard X-rays can only detect bone loss after it is in this advanced stage. Fortunately, more sensitive screening tests that can more accurately predict the early onset of osteoporosis are now widely available. In particular, dual-energy X-ray absorptiometry (DEXA) uses low-dose X-ray to assess bone density in the lower spine and hip, the sites of most osteoporotic fractures. If this test result shows lowered density, additional blood and urine tests are generally called for.

Unfortunately, even the best tests measure only bone density, not brittleness. Bones that are flexible, despite having less mass, will resist fracture. Thus, while DEXA can give clues to current levels of bone density in the bones measured, women should take note of early osteoporosis warning signs, such as periodontal disease, changes in the curvature of the spinal column leading to "dowager's hump," and unrelenting back pains. While several new drugs have been developed that appear to reduce the rate of fracture, the key to long-term bone health remains prevention.

BARE BONES: THE FACTS ON YOUR BONES AND OSTEOPOROSIS

Let's start with our bones themselves. It may not seem like it, but bone is living tissue, made primarily of calcium, but also of other essential minerals and protein. We have two types of bone in our bodies: compact bone, which is found in the shafts of long bones because it is able to withstand tensile stress, and trabecular bone, which is more weight-efficient and is found in heel bones, vertebrae, and the end of long bone shafts. Compact bone looks solid and hard, while spongy bone is like its name, spongy and filled with holes. Within both types of bone are two groups of bone cells; one type, osteoclasts, breaks down old bone and the other, osteoblasts, is responsible for making new bone. This breaking down and rebuilding process is called remodeling and takes place throughout our lifetime. The "turnover" time for compact bone is approximately ten to twelve years; the turnover time for trabecular bone can be as short as two to three years.

Anywhere from 5 to 10 percent of our bone is replaced every year by this remodeling process. From childhood until our early 20s—depending on sex, race, exercise levels, nutrition, and overall health—bone is made faster than it is broken down, resulting in the formation of dense, healthy bones. According to the peak bone mass concept, by our early 20s our bones reach their peak of perfection. The greater the bone mass we achieve by this point in our lives, the less our risk of osteoporosis later. Therefore, prevention of this crippling disease begins in childhood and adolescence with proper nutrition.

By our late 30s and early 40s, the balance of bone growth and loss begins to change and a slow, steady decline in total bone mass begins. Age-related bone loss seems to be normal, but rapid or accelerated loss of bone results in osteoporosis. Bones become weakened and brittle. The walls of compact bone become thinner and softer, and the holes in the spongy bone become larger, leading to a greater risk of fractures and breaks. While the rate and amount of bone thinning varies widely among individuals, generally among women bone loss begins in their mid-20s and accelerates four or five years after menopause.

THE CAUSES OF OSTEOPOROSIS

Like menopause, osteoporosis is not a hormone-deficiency disease, and the primary treatment should not be hormone replacement therapy (HRT). Nevertheless, sex steroid, thyroid, and parathyroid hormones have major roles to play in the bone-remodeling process.

The Role of Estrogen

Before you reach menopause, estrogen helps control the bone-destroying osteoclasts. The estrogen pushes your thyroid to produce calcitonin, which increases calcium uptake by bones. Then you reach menopause. The estrogen/progesterone imbalance that occurs during this time allows the osteoclasts to increase the rate of bone loss, thus accelerating osteoporosis. As levels of various other hormones diminish during menopause, the absorption of calcium and magnesium by the bone also decreases. However, no definitive studies have been published showing that lower levels of estrogen cause osteoporosis, so there is no justification for prescribing HRT to prevent it. At least one major study found that after seven years of menopause, the decline in bone mineral density was the same whether women were on HRT or not. In addition, other research has shown that just as much bone is lost when estrogen therapy is interrupted or stopped as would have been lost if it had never been started. And as discussed in Chapter 1, the dangerous association of HRT with varying degrees of increased risk of breast cancer, blood clotting, stroke, heart disease, and dementia makes it an undesirable treatment for osteoporosis or other menopausal symptoms.

Doctors often ignore the fact that many other factors contribute to the risk of developing osteoporosis, including past and present amounts of calcium and other bone-building minerals and vitamins in your diet; your ability to absorb these important nutrients; past and present exercise levels; and dietary and lifestyle habits. An apt analogy can be made with an automobile. When a car begins using too much oil, we know better than to blame the oil. Lack of proper maintenance, regular oil changes, and tune-ups over the years has led to this problem. We can continue to drive the automobile and pour oil into it to keep it functioning and risk further damage by just treating the symptom, or we can take it to the auto mechanic and get to the root of the problem. Perhaps we'll need a complete engine overhaul, a balancing, if you will, of the pistons, rings, and valves. Similarly, if we have carefully maintained our bodies over the years with proper diet and exercise, our bodies will be in balance and our declining estrogen levels will not create the severe problems we have been told to expect. Adding more "oil" in the form of estrogen will not cure the problems and may put us at greater risk of other, more serious health problems.

The Role of Other Sex Hormones

The connection between progesterone and osteoporosis has been grossly overlooked. One of the major physiological effects of progesterone is to stimulate new bone formation. This is particularly important during menopause, when decreased progesterone levels alone can cause rapid bone loss. Unfortunately, many women arrive at menopause with a profound progesterone deficiency due to adrenal exhaustion (see Chapter 2). Natural progesterone body cream may be quite helpful in restoring hormonal balance to the system before menopause occurs, thereby preventing bone-thinning.

Both testosterone and dehydroepiandrosterone (DHEA) have been shown to promote bone growth. Unfortunately, levels of both decline with age—after menopause, testosterone levels, for example, are about half what they were before menopause. While results are inconclu-sive, some research has found a strong enough correlation between the decline in DHEA levels and bone density to suggest a possible use as a diagnostic indicator.

Interplay of Endocrine Hormones

Our bodies have developed a highly complex system to ensure we have a sound skeleton and enough circulating calcium to meet its needs. The thyroid gland produces one hormone (calcitonin) that pushes the os-teoblasts to build new bone. This process, of course, removes calcium from the blood. Another thyroid hormone (thyroxine, or T4) does the opposite, having its effect on the osteoclasts to break down old bone.

Sensing when blood calcium levels are low, another gland, the parathyroid, produces yet another hormone, parathyroid hormone (PTH), which breaks down bone to replenish the blood calcium. High calcium levels cause PTH to increase calcium absorption by bone, boost calcium excretion by the kidneys, and decrease phosphate ab-sorption, so the phosphates can bind with excess calcium to make it biologically unavailable. Thus, anything that interferes with any step in this process can lead to osteoporosis. Women with hypothyroidism who take thyroxine will lose bone mineral, particularly from the spine. Hyperthyroidism also increases the risk of osteoporosis.

RISK FACTORS FOR OSTEOPOROSIS

Living to a ripe old age is sure to result in some loss of bone tissue. But not everyone—and not even every woman who goes through menopause and lives with reduced estrogen levels—develops osteo-porosis. Certain hereditary factors have been identified that increase the likelihood of developing osteoporosis; these are things over which we have no control at the present time.

While both men and women develop osteoporosis, women are at greater risk. Women's bones are lighter and smaller, and a greater proportion of their total bone is lost as compared with men. Women are also at greater risk because bone loss occurs much more rapidly as estrogen levels decrease. If you experience menopause earlier in life, your estrogen levels are reduced over a longer period of time, and your risk of developing osteoporosis is greater. If you are thin and short and have a small frame and small bones, you're at greater risk because you have less body fat stores and therefore produce less estrogen after menopause than do heavier women.

Osteoporosis is more common among whites, especially of northern European descent, and Asians. Black women have a lower risk because their bones are normally larger and they lose bone mass more slowly. If you have a mother, grandmother, sister, or aunt who has developed osteoporosis, you are more likely to develop it, too. Certain diseases—including endocrine disorders, diabetes, and arthritis—also put you at greater risk. In addition to these hereditary factors, certain lifestyle habits increase your risk of developing osteoporosis. These things we do have control over, and with the Hot Times approach, we can take steps to change our habits and increase our chances of living a long and healthy life.

A Note About Medication

While some medications prescribed by your doctor are necessary, excessive use of certain drugs may lead to osteoporosis because of calcium loss. Diuretics like Lasix, corticosteroids, excess thyroid medication, and prolonged antibiotic use often deplete the body's store of calcium. If you are currently taking any of these medications, you should take extra steps to ensure that your calcium level is maintained.

CALCIUM: SEPARATING FACT FROM FICTION

Next to hot flashes, osteoporosis is perhaps the condition most associated with menopause and aging in women. Hidden beneath our skin, our bones are silently and often painlessly becoming less dense and more fragile. It's a frightening prospect indeed. But there's a simple, relatively inexpensive, harmless way to prevent osteoporosis: just take calcium. At least that's what the dairy, processed food, and dietary supplement industries would have us believe. Calcium has been added to breakfast cereals, orange juice, and canned soups; it even comes in fudgelike squares. Women's magazines and television advertisements promote it; doctors recommend it to their patients.

Calcium is so important to our bodies that Mother Nature has produced a complex system to ensure we maintain optimum levels. Blood levels must stay between 9 and 11 mg of calcium per 100 cc of blood. When our intake of calcium is too low to maintain this level and blood calcium levels drop, parathyroid hormone dissolves calcium from our bones to resupply the blood.

In addition to its vital role in forming and maintaining strong bones and teeth, calcium is the key mineral for maintaining muscle tone and elasticity. It is needed for muscle growth and contraction, and it delays the onset of muscle fatigue and increases stamina— including for the heart. Calcium can even help lower blood pressure in certain individuals by helping relax the smooth muscle of the peripheral blood vessels. Calcium is also necessary for the absorption of vitamin B_{12}, which keeps our nerves healthy. In addition, calcium works on the nervous system, playing an important role in the transmission of nerve impulses from one part of our bodies to another, "nourishing" the nerves and exhibiting a sedative effect on the nervous system. Circulating calcium helps blood clot, and calcium metabolism has been shown to play a role in lessening hypertension.

But despite all these benefits of calcium, the "take calcium" messages gloss over one important point: too much calcium can have serious health consequences for women. By too much calcium, I refer not only to taking much more than your body can store and use, but also to factors that cause the calcium you ingest to be biologically unavailable. You need to absorb about 600 mg of calcium each day for optimum bone-building, but after menopause you may absorb less than 7 percent of the calcium you take.

Unlike other minerals, excess calcium is not immediately and fully excreted through the kidneys. While bones and teeth are primary storage sites, more excess calcium accumulates in joints, contributing to arthritis, and in your blood vessels. Calcified plaques form along the vessel walls, contributing to high blood pressure and blockages that could lead to a heart attack. Research has found a strong correlation between calcium deposits in your arteries and the presence of equally artery-clogging fatty plaques. Calcium that accumulates in your aorta causes it to lose its flexibility, and if in your heart muscle, it can lead to an irregular heartbeat, known as arrhythmia. Excess calcium can also accumulate in your kidneys, leading to kidney stones.

The Effect of Diet on Calcium Absorption

If calcium absorption and excretion are to be balanced, your body needs optimum levels of numerous cofactors, in particular magnesium, but also boron; copper; manganese; silicon; zinc; and vitamins B_6, B_{12}, C, D, and K and folic acid. We'll look more closely at each of these in a moment. First, let's see how choices you make in your diet affect how much calcium reaches your bones.

The typical American diet is high in the wrong kind of fat, sugar, sodium, and phosphorus, all of which cause problems with calcium absorption and utilization. Excess saturated fats, such as those found in full-fat dairy products (such as cheese and ice cream), pork, beef, and the tropical oils (including palm, palm kernel, and coconut), combine with calcium in the intestines, forming insoluble compounds and rendering the calcium unusable. Excess sodium causes calcium to be excreted in the urine. This in turn lowers blood levels of calcium, signaling your hormone system to cause calcium to be withdrawn from your bones to maintain the proper blood calcium level.

Women who follow dietary recommendations for eating a low-protein, high complex-carbohydrate diet containing heavy whole grains in the form of wheat, rye, oats, barley, and bran may unwittingly create a calcium absorption problem as well. Grains contain phytic acid, a phosphorus-like compound that combines with calcium in the intestine and blocks its absorption. In excess (as in some vegetarian diets), grains can also provide too much insoluble fiber. An overabundance of insoluble fiber can interfere with the absorption of minerals such as calcium, zinc, and manganese. Fiber binds with these minerals and carries them out of the body unused. Daily excess consumption of food containing oxalic acid can also interfere with calcium absorption. The oxalic acid found in cooked spinach, chard, beet and dandelion greens, sorrel, rhubarb, asparagus, and chocolate binds with calcium to form calcium oxalate, which is indigestible and can cause kidney stones in some individuals.

THE HOT TIMES APPROACH TO OSTEOPOROSIS

There's much more to preventing osteoporosis than eating dairy products and taking large doses of calcium supplements. If you have read this far, you realize that, over time, our bodies have developed a delicately balanced system for building and protecting our bones. The plan I follow and recommend to my clients includes the following steps:

- Eliminate "calcium robbers"—sugar, soda, caffeine, processed foods, aluminum, and too much saturated fat, complex carbohydrates and grains, and oxalic acid—as much as possible.
- Choose food sources described in this chapter (instead of relying on dairy) to supply most of your calcium needs and to provide vital vitamin and mineral bone nutrients. As much as possible, use whole foods, organically grown, and avoid overcooking to retain nutrients. Chapter 8 offers a wonderful selection of recipes to help you incorporate a wide range of healthful foods in your menu planning.
- Take appropriate supplements. Although we should try to obtain our calcium and other bone-building nutrients from our diets, this is becoming more and more difficult. Modern agricultural methods have left us with a legacy of poor soil. Minerals that were once abundant in our soil, and consequently in our food, have been depleted. Those that remain are often removed in processing, shipping, or exposure to light.

Dietary Dangers: The Calcium Robbers

It's so easy to add calcium to your diet, it's not surprising really that so many of you have already done so. I admit it's a bit harder to get control of all the calcium robbers you consume, but it's essential if you're to benefit from the calcium in your diet. My Hot Times approach, including many of the recipes, makes it easier to leave these robbers behind.

SUGAR: THE ULTIMATE CALCIUM ROBBER

Sugar may be the number-one cause of calcium imbalance. In order for calcium to be transported to bone marrow, it needs to be in balance with phosphorus. According to Melvin Page, D.D.S., a pioneer researcher in dental endocrinology, a healthy calcium-phosphorus level is 2.5 parts calcium to 1 part phosphorus. Without adequate phosphorus for transport, bone marrow doesn't get the calcium it needs, so the body pulls calcium from storage sites in bone. But this acquired calcium cannot be used without adequate phosphorus, and results in an "excess" of calcium that is ultimately just excreted from the body. Eventually, this imbalance of calcium and phosphorus starves the bone marrow of calcium, resulting in osteoporosis.

Because sugar depletes your body of phosphorus, eating sugar can profoundly disturb your calcium-phosphorus ratio, despite your intake of calcium. In the process of being metabolized, refined sugars also rob the body of other valuable nutrients, including magnesium, manganese, chromium, zinc, copper, and cobalt, thereby causing an imbalance in all the body's minerals. This imbalance contributes not only to osteoporosis but to other degenerative diseases as well, including heart disease and diabetes.

Today you will probably eat 45 teaspoons of sugar. While you would never willfully eat spoonfuls of sugar straight out of the sugar bowl, this is actually the equivalent of the combined amount of sugar found in a 12-ounce glass of fruit punch, a 12-ounce can of Mountain Dew, and two 8-ounce containers of low-fat fruit yogurt. All of this adds up to about 170 pounds of sugar for the average American every year.

I can hear many of you protesting, "I don't eat sugar anymore. I'm eating more fiber, and I've cut out desserts." But everything, from cigarettes to french fries, has sugar in it. Low-fat fruit yogurt has 13 teaspoons and even pickled beets contain almost 10 teaspoons per serving. Food preparers have discovered that sugar is not just for sweetening. Added to foods such as catsup, it helps retain colors; added to baked goods, it ferments yeast and imparts a brown crust to breads and rolls; in soft drinks it adds body and texture; in chewing gum, pliability. Molasses or corn syrup may be added to a restaurant's hamburgers, and raw potato slices are often dipped in sugared water before being fried.

Remember, too, sugar is more than the white granulated stuff we put in our coffee. There are more than a dozen other kinds from a variety of sources, including glucose, fructose, maltose, lactose, dextrose, raw sugar, honey, brown sugar, powdered sugar, molasses, maple sugar, corn syrup, high-fructose corn syrup, rice syrup, and barley malt. Also, sorbitol, mannitol, and xylitol are sugar alcohols. These sugars are hidden in an abundant variety of our foods. When "choosy mothers choose Jif" peanut butter, they're also choosing sugar. And if you're eating Lipton Cup-a-Soup, Ritz crackers, Hellmann's mayonnaise, Quaker Instant Oatmeal, Gatorade, bacon, hot dogs, bologna, nondairy creamers, or cream-style corn, you're getting a strong dose of sugar. Chewing gum contains one-half teaspoon per stick. We pat ourselves on the back for switching from a sugar-coated cereal to Fruit & Fibre, not realizing that it contains 46 percent sugar per half-cup serving. Although much of that sugar occurs naturally in the raisins, malt, and grains, the negative effects of sugar on calcium seem to be the same no matter which form you consume.

Food labels are the key to controlling our sugar habits. Read those colorful paper labels carefully and search for any of the "-ose" words (glucose, dextrose, sucrose, etc.). Sugar will also be listed as corn syrup, honey, molasses, barley malt, or just sweetener. To reduce sugar in your day-to-day diet, you may want to:

- Make your own muffins, puddings, gelatins, sorbets, and fruit desserts so you can control the sugar content. In general, you can cut back on the amount of sugar called for in a recipe by one-third to one-half without affecting taste.
- Drink unsweetened fruit juice mixed half and half with mineral water or seltzer instead of regular or diet soft drinks. You can also drink 100 percent fruit juice.
- Use fresh fruit as snacks or desserts—but don't go overboard. Although fruit is rich in fiber, vitamins, and minerals, it is also high in natural sugars.
- Avoid using sweets as rewards, either for yourself or your family. More than any other food, sweets become entangled in our psychological and emotional lives; we celebrate with cake, we

console ourselves with Häagen-Dazs. Learn your own triggers and work at breaking the habit. Keep a food diary to help you pinpoint when you tend to rely on sugar to improve your mood.

SODA AND SOFT DRINKS:
CREATING UNBALANCE

Sodas are the nation's number-one drink; more soda is consumed than even water. Most sodas not only contain sugar, they also contain large amounts of phosphoric acid, a phosphorus-containing substance. While some phosphorus is necessary for bone and calcium metabolism, its presence in meat, other protein foods, and artificially preserved foods, in addition to soft drinks, causes us to consume much more phosphorus than calcium and creates an imbalance between these nutrients. Since the ratio of phosphorus to calcium in our bodies is a critical factor in the optimal use of calcium, drinking soft drinks throws this ratio entirely out of whack.

Adding more calcium to your diet would seem to be a way to bring this ratio back into balance. But when we take in high levels of calcium, the body actually absorbs it at lower levels while continuing to absorb phosphorus efficiently. High levels of both have been shown to lead to the loss of other important minerals in the body. Over the past several decades, our intake of phosphorus has doubled while our calcium intake has declined. This may be due to the fact that even though we may be taking calcium supplements, we're doing other things that inhibit calcium absorption. Some research suggests that phosphorus from nonessential sources, including sodas and soft drinks and artificially preserved foods, may be more detrimental to the calcium/phosphorus ratio than phosphorus occurring in meat and other protein foods.

So many of us have fallen into a destructive cycle: drinking soda, which depletes our calcium, and then megadosing on calcium supplements in an effort to restore calcium levels, which leads to further loss. We would do well to eliminate all sources of nonessential phosphorus from our diets. Certain mineral waters are good substitutes for soda and soft drinks, providing us with additional calcium but no sugar. For example, six 8-ounce glasses of imported waters, such as S. Pellegrino and Vittel Grande Source, provide 1200 mg of calcium.

CAFFEINE: NOTORIOUS CALCIUM DEPLETER

Lattes, cappuccinos, and espressos are morning treats, and necessities to some, that many of us enjoy every day. But that gourmet coffee you start your morning off with is sucking the calcium from your bones. Caffeine is a powerful diuretic, doubling the rate at which calcium leaves your body in urine. The excretion of calcium stimulates the parathyroid gland to secrete the hormone responsible for drawing more calcium from the bone to replace it in the bloodstream. In addition, coffee contains twenty-nine different acids, which draw even more calcium from the bone to act as a neutralizer.

Excessive consumption of coffee, tea, regular soft drinks, chocolate, and other foods containing caffeine (see Table 3-1 below) will in-

Table 3-1 Foods and Beverages Containing Caffeine

Product	Caffeine (average mg)
Coffee (5 oz)	
Brewed, drip method	80
Instant	65
Decaffeinated, brewed	3
Decaffeinated, instant	2
Tea (5 oz)	
Brewed, major U.S. brands	40
Brewed, imported brands	60
Instant	30
Iced (12 oz), brewed	70
Cocoa (5 oz)	4
Chocolate milk (8 oz)	5
Dark chocolate, semisweet (1 oz)	6
Baker's chocolate (1 oz)	26
Chocolate-flavored syrup (1 oz)	4

Reprinted from *Healthy Bones*, by Nancy Appleton, Ph.D. Published by Avery Publishing Group, Inc., Garden City Park, New York. Used with permission.

crease your risk for osteoporosis by reducing blood calcium levels, triggering calcium to be pulled from bone and flushing needed calcium out of your body. And it doesn't take much to be excessive. A mere three cups of black coffee a day can result in a 45-mg calcium loss. Unfortunately, women between the ages of 35 and 50, who often need calcium the most, drink more coffee than any other age group.

You're not any better off drinking carbonated soft drinks (see Table 3-2). The combination of caffeine and sugar may actually increase the loss of calcium through the urine more than when either of the two is used alone. In addition to coffee, tea, soft drinks, and chocolate, many prescription and nonprescription drugs contain caffeine. According to FDA figures, more than a thousand over-the-

Table 3-2 Caffeine Content of Soft Drinks

Product	Caffeine (mg per 12-oz serving)
Carbonated	
Cherry Coke, Coca-Cola	46
Cherry cola, Slice	48
Cherry RC	36
Coca-Cola	46
Coca-Cola Classic	46
Cola	37
Cola, RC	36
Mello Yello	52
Mr. Pibb	40
Mountain Dew	54
Dr Pepper–type soda	37
Pepsi	38
Carbonated, low-calorie	
Diet Cherry Coke, Coca-Cola	46
Diet Cherry Cola, Slice	48
Diet Coke, Coca-Cola	46
Diet cola, aspartame-sweetened	50
Diet Pepsi	36
Diet RC	48
Tab	46

Reprinted from *Healthy Bones*, by Nancy Appleton, Ph.D. Published by Avery Publishing Group, Inc., Garden City Park, New York. Used with permission.

counter drugs have caffeine as one of their ingredients. These include cold medicines, pain relievers, weight-control products, and allergy remedies. As with sugar, in some cases we are unknowingly ingesting caffeine.

PHOSPHORUS: TOO MUCH OF A GOOD THING

As discussed above, in order for calcium to be transported to bone marrow, it needs to be in balance with phosphorus. But the typical American diet is relatively low in calcium and high in phosphorus. Too much meat, poultry, nuts, seeds, seafood, whole grains, and soft drinks wreak havoc with the body's calcium-phosphorus ratio because these foods are much higher in phosphorus than calcium to begin with. Meats such as ham or pork chops contain up to thirty times more phosphorus than calcium; chicken contains more phosphorus (250 mg in 3.5 oz) than even lean cuts of red meat (158 mg in 3.5 oz of ground lean beef). High-phosphorus foods, including cow's milk, cause calcium to form insoluble compounds that lead to inadequate absorption of any calcium consumed. Phosphorus is also found in many of the convenience foods we've grown to rely on in our busy lives, like processed cheese, baked goods containing phosphate baking powder, puddings, bread, and instant soups.

ALUMINUM: THE HIDDEN CALCIUM ROBBER

You probably haven't realized it, but aluminum—often contained in antacids, buffered aspirins, and foods—is a calcium robber. Ordinarily, you may consume about 20 mg aluminum every day, but many popular antacids (Maalox, Amphojel, Gelusil, Mylanta) contain from 35 to 208 mg of aluminum per tablet. Buffered aspirin, depending upon the particular brand, can deliver an extra 10 to 52 mg of aluminum per tablet. You should avoid eating foods cooked in aluminum pans or wrapped in foil, beverages served in aluminum cans, processed cheeses, cheese spreads, cream cheese, pickled foods, some nonprescription drugs with high aluminum content, and peppermint tea. Aluminum-containing antacids, taken three to four times a day for two to five weeks, have been shown to inhibit absorption of phosphorus. While too much phosphorus creates a problem with calcium utilization, too little phosphorus is just as detrimental. Remember, it's the balance that's crucial.

Getting the Calcium You Need

Now that you've given up coffee and soda, and cut down on your sugar, where are you going to get your calcium? The dairy industry has not been shy in telling us that dairy products contain abundant calcium. The vast majority of us grew up knowing that milk builds strong bones and healthy teeth. Indeed, most of us were raised on milk and still look to it and other dairy products as good sources of calcium. We, as a nation, consume more dairy products than any other, yet we still have more calcium-related degenerative diseases—including osteoporosis, osteoarthritis, arteriosclerosis, and cataracts—than nations where dairy consumption is minimal or nonexistent. In Asia and Africa, areas where milk products are not included in the diet, the incidence of osteoporosis is negligible, while in Europe and North America, where milk and milk products are heavily consumed, osteoporosis is reaching epidemic proportions. What's going on?

The answer to this question is that Americans mainly rely on milk and milk products to get calcium in their diets. Yes, milk is rich in calcium—1200 mg per quart to be exact, more than enough to satisfy a whole day's requirement. But it's almost equally rich in phosphorus, the mineral that we have already discussed with the biochemical bad habit of interfering with calcium absorption. Milk's high phosphorus content (the ratio is 1.2 parts calcium to 1 part phosphorus) impairs calcium absorption. Infants drinking mother's milk, which contains only 300 mg of calcium per quart but has a beneficial calcium-phosphorus ratio of 2:1, actually absorb more calcium than infants drinking cows' milk. Milk and milk products also tend to neutralize hydrochloric acid in the stomach and generate excessive mucus in the intestines. Both of these factors interfere with the proper absorption of calcium.

Milk also has nearly ten times more calcium than magnesium, which puts yet another strain on your body's ability to absorb calcium. Magnesium helps calcium absorption, but too much calcium interferes with the absorption of magnesium. Magnesium reduces the body's need for calcium, but calcium increases the body's need for magnesium. Although this may seem confusing, humans evolved in a magnesium-rich, calcium-poor environment. Our bodies, therefore, learned to conserve calcium but not magnesium. To correct this imbalance, it makes good sense to favor magnesium-rich foods in our diets over foods like milk that are high in calcium. Read more about this vital mineral seesaw later in this chapter.

Finally, for the majority of the world's adult population, milk is a source of calcium they cannot biochemically utilize. At some point between the ages of 18 months and 4 years, most people stop producing the intestinal enzyme called lactase that is needed to break down milk sugar, or lactose. This normal process is similar to that in the animal world, where the lactase enzyme becomes unnecessary shortly after weaning. The resulting lack of lactase causes undigested lactose to move into the colon, where it ferments, resulting in bloating, gas, cramps, and, in some cases, diarrhea. Humans are the only animals that continue to drink milk after weaning, yet worldwide, far more people suffer from lactose intolerance than do not, and therefore cannot benefit from the calcium in milk.

Milk: A Source of Calcium . . . and Fat

While advertisers have focused our attention on the calcium in milk, they have neglected to honestly inform us about its fat content. Milk can be high in saturated fat, which has been

implicated in cardiovascular disease. The milk industry decep-
tively reports fat content by weight rather than by calories.
While whole milk is labeled 3.5 percent fat by weight, which
seems acceptable, 49 percent of its calories actually are from
fat—which is outrageous.

The truth is that there are better dietary sources of calcium available that will ensure balanced nutrient levels in your body and maxi-
mize calcium absorption and utilization. Whether you get your calcium
from food or supplements, it will be largely ineffective without various cofactors. These include minerals, especially magnesium, and
several vitamins. Each has a role to play in ensuring your bones stay
strong and healthy. Some minerals, such as magnesium, work directly
on bone cells to give flexibility and strength. Others, including copper and manganese, help produce the enzymes needed to make collagen, a component of your connective tissue. Whatever their action,
the minerals discussed below are commonly deficient in modern diets, so my multifaceted Hot Times approach brings you into balance.

NONDAIRY SOURCES OF CALCIUM

Despite what the dairy lobby would have you believe, numerous
other foods are rich in calcium—and they are balanced in their phosphorus or magnesium levels, which ensures that the calcium actually
gets used. More calcium can be found in a cup of cooked collard
greens than in a cup of milk, and 2 tablespoons of good old-fashioned
blackstrap molasses have almost the same amount of calcium as a
cup of milk.

Interestingly, although chocolate does not have much calcium,
one-quarter cup of carob flour, a healthy chocolate substitute, contains a respectable 120 mg of this bone-building mineral. Herbs rich
in calcium include nettle, dandelion greens, watercress, and chick-

weed. Sea vegetables such as hijiki, wakame, and kombu are also good sources; one-half cup of cooked hijiki is almost as high in calcium as one-half cup of milk. Table 3-3 gives you many other choices for your daily diet, and the recipes in Chapter 8 include even more creative ways to get calcium and bone-building nutrients from your meals.

If you use soy products as dairy substitutes, remember that tofu is calcium-rich only when calcium sulfate has been added for coagulation. Similarly, soy milk, unless it has been fortified with extra calcium, is not a substantial calcium source. And as discussed in Chapter 1, unfermented soy products contain phytoestrogens, which can interfere with your estrogen-progesterone balance.

CALCIUM SUPPLEMENTS

The form of supplemental calcium I recommend is microcrystalline hydroxyapatite (MCHC), because research has shown it to be among the best-absorbed of the various calcium compounds. It appears MCHC not only stops bone loss but also regenerates bone. Other absorbable forms of calcium include calcium citrate, calcium aspartate, calcium succinate, and calcium ascorbate. You will want to look for supplements that include these forms of calcium as well as magnesium. The brand OsteoKey from Uni Key Health Systems provides calcium and magnesium in a 1:1 ratio, along with other bone-building vitamins and trace minerals.

The Daily Reference Intake value for calcium is 1200 mg for women over 50, but given the negative health consequences of excess calcium, I question the need for such high amounts. Recent studies also indicate that high levels of calcium don't actually improve bone density. Researchers from the Mayo Clinic, for example, found the rate of bone loss to be the same for women taking 1400 mg calcium daily and another group taking just 500 mg. Depending upon how much calcium you are getting in your foods, I recommend anywhere from 250 to 1000 mg per day of additional calcium from dietary supplements.

Table 3-3 Nondairy Calcium Sources

Food/substance	Mg/100 g edible portion (100 g = 3.5 oz)
Kelp	1093
Carob flour	352
Dulse	296
Collard leaves	250
Turnip greens	248
Barbados molasses	245
Almonds	234
Brewer's yeast	210
Parsley	203
Corn tortillas, lime added	200
Dandelion greens	187
Brazil nuts	186
Watercress	151
Goats' milk	129
Tofu	128
Dried figs	126
Sunflower seeds	120
Wheat bran	119
Buckwheat, raw	114
Sesame seeds, hulled	110
Ripe olives	106
Broccoli	103
English walnut	99
Spinach (raw)	93
Soybeans, cooked	73
Pecans	73
Wheat germ	72
Peanuts	69
Miso	68
Romaine lettuce	68
Dried apricots (unsulfured)	67
Rutabaga	66
Raisins	62
Black currants	60
Dates	59
Green snap beans	58
Globe artichoke	51
Dried prunes	51
Pumpkin and squash seeds	51
Cooked dry beans	50

Data from Endo-met Laboratories, Phoenix, Arizona, based on evaluation of existing literature.

When you do look for a calcium supplement, keep in mind that while most manufacturers list the total amount of calcium compound provided in each tablet on the label, this number doesn't indicate the amount of elemental calcium—that is, the amount of calcium actually available to your body. The amount of elemental calcium in each tablet depends on the compound used. Following is a list of the most common supplements and the percent of elemental calcium in each:

- calcium carbonate: 40 percent
- hydroxyapatite: 30 percent
- calcium citrate: 24 percent
- calcium lactate: 13 percent
- calcium gluconate: 9 percent

So if you are taking calcium carbonate (40 percent elemental calcium) and the label says each tablet contains 1000 mg, you are actually getting only 400 mg of elemental calcium; the rest is carbonate.

Several other compounds are relatively good sources of elemental calcium but should be avoided. Avoid taking calcium phosphate, as our diets are already too high in phosphorus. You should also avoid bonemeal and dolomite, because they may be contaminated with lead, toxic minerals, and pesticides.

If you are experiencing symptoms of magnesium deficiency—such as extreme edginess, muscle cramps or tremors, apathy, sleeping problems, or increased urination—consider adjusting your calcium-magnesium intake so you are taking twice as much magnesium as calcium. Take 500 to 1000 mg of magnesium at a different time of day from when you take a calcium supplement, and avoid taking the magnesium with meals, because it neutralizes stomach acids that you need for digestion and calcium absorption. Once you feel a better balance has been achieved, return to the 1:1 ratio of calcium and magnesium. If you experience diarrhea, reduce your magne-

sium intake. If you have kidney disease, do not take magnesium supplements.

If you get adequate calcium from your diet and don't need a high-
dose calcium supplement, you may want to consider taking a high-
quality multiple vitamin supplement that includes all the vitamin and
mineral bone nutrients discussed in this chapter. For example, the
Female Multiple from Uni Key Health Systems (800-888-4353) has
just 250 mg calcium but 500 mg magnesium; the formula meets or
exceeds the recommended levels of the other vitamins and minerals
needed to keep your bones healthy and is free of copper and phosphorus, which tend to be excessive in our diets.

Dietary Recommendations

Osteoporosis, perhaps more so than any other female condition, is a
telltale sign of how you've been living your life over the past twenty to
thirty years. While often the result of genetics, it can also be a natural consequence of what you've been eating, how you've been exercising, your consumption of coffee and sodas, and those high-protein
or high-carbohydrate diets you followed from time to time. Although
many sources claim that absorption of calcium in the intestine typically diminishes with age, leaving us helpless against osteoporosis, I
do not believe this to be inevitable but simply yet another consequence of a lifetime of poor nutritional habits.

MAGNESIUM
With all the focus on calcium for building strong, healthy bones,
the significance of magnesium has virtually been ignored, but that is
changing. In 2003, for example, Mildred S. Seelig, M.D., MPH, and
Andrea Rosanoff, Ph.D., published *The Magnesium Factor,* which
should help bring this mineral's essential nature to a broad audience.

Where calcium causes muscles to contract, magnesium causes

them to relax. Calcium stimulates nerves, and magnesium calms them by slowing the release of epinephrine and norepinephrine by the adrenal glands. Calcium is essential for blood clotting, but magnesium keeps blood flowing freely and prevents abnormal coagulation. I'll talk more about the role of magnesium in heart health in the next chapter, but for now, I want to focus on the calcium-magnesium relationship and its impact on your bones.

Magnesium is a component of every cell membrane. In your bones, magnesium is found within the soft bone matrix, where it gives bones flexibility. When magnesium levels are low, bones become brittle and subject to fracture. To compensate for this, when levels of magnesium are low, calcium can enter cells to help keep them strong. But if calcium levels rise significantly within cells, the cells harden—a process known as calcification.

In order for your body to keep blood calcium levels stable, the parathyroid gland produces parathyroid hormone (PTH), which causes calcium to be drawn from bone when blood calcium levels are low. Another hormone, calcitonin, stimulates calcium deposits within bone. Magnesium suppresses the action of PTH and stimulates calcitonin, thus building bone density. A study by Guy E. Abraham, M.D., and Harinder Grewal published in the *Journal of Reproductive Medicine* found that postmenopausal women who took just 500 mg of calcium with 600 to 1000 mg of magnesium had an average increase in bone density of 11 percent within a year. Magnesium also helps prevent formation of kidney stones (calcium oxalate crystals), and it is needed to convert vitamin D to its active form so that calcium can be absorbed into the bone. Thus, magnesium helps bones two ways: by providing flexibility and by adding density.

Unfortunately, current tests are unreliable in determining levels of magnesium in your body. However, there are many dietary practices that can contribute to magnesium deficiency. A diet rich in sugar, caffeinated beverages, or excess alcohol will cause you to excrete magnesium in your urine, causing deficiency. Also, saturated fat and phosphorus, found in soft drinks and many processed foods, block magnesium absorption. And omitting leafy green vegetables, nuts, seeds, or sea vegetables from your diet can also cause magnesium deficiency.

There are a number of lifestyle indicators of magnesium deficiency as well. If you crave chocolate, your body may actually be crying out for magnesium, since cocoa powder is one of the richest sources of magnesium. But, sorry, a Hershey bar doesn't qualify as a healthful magnesium food source! If you are under a lot of physical or mental stress, the hormones your adrenal glands produce in response to stress increase magnesium excretion. Also, diuretics, certain antibiotics, digitalis, and HRT, all either increase magnesium excretion or your body's need for the mineral. A number of menopausal symptoms may in fact be signs of magnesium deficiency, including irritability, memory loss, concentration problems, depression, sleep difficulties, muscle cramps, and increased urination. Extreme edginess is a telltale symptom of magnesium deficiency.

The Daily Reference Intake level for magnesium is 320 mg for women 50 and older, which you can get from a diet rich in leafy green vegetables, kale, celery, alfalfa sprouts, beans, seeds, and nuts. But as the typical American consumes only about 100 mg daily, I suggest supplementing your food sources with additional magnesium (see page 81).

BORON

It wasn't until the mid-1980s that researchers began uncovering what it is that boron contributes to our health. Like calcium, boron is found primarily in our bones and teeth and appears to have a role in bone health, particularly for menopausal women. A study at the U.S. Department of Agriculture found that after eight days of 3-mg supplements of boron, postmenopausal women lost 40 percent less calcium, 33 percent less magnesium, and slightly less phosphorus than those not taking the supplements. The study also concluded that

Table 3-4 Boron Content of Foods

Food	Boron Content (mg)
1 g prunes (unsulfured)	27
1 g raisins (unsulfured)	25
1 g almonds	23
1 g peanuts	18
1 g hazelnuts	16
1 g dates (unsulfured)	9.2
1 g honey	7.2
1 medium apple	1
1½ cups apple sauce	1
2½ cups grape juice	1
Based on evaluation of existing literature.	

boron is necessary for the synthesis of estrogen and vitamin D. Another study has shown that supplementation of boron raised serum estrogen levels of postmenopausal women not on estrogen replacement therapy to levels comparable to those of women receiving estrogen.

As an essential trace element, boron is necessary to our well-being, but we need only small amounts of it each day. At present, no Daily Reference Intake level for boron has been determined, but it appears that 1 to 2 mg of boron a day can meet your body's needs. Boron is found in plant foods, especially fruits (fresh or dried), vegetables, nuts, and honey. Table 3-4 lists the boron content of some common foods. As long as you eat a moderate amount of these foods every day, you'll easily get a healthy, bone-building level of boron in your body.

COPPER

Copper is essential for the production of an enzyme needed to form collagen and elastin, the proteins that provide the basic material for your connective tissues, cartilage, and bone. Few of us are technically deficient in copper today; rather we are copper-toxic, because of excessive copper accumulation in our brain, liver, and other organs. When copper accumulates in these soft tissues, it becomes biologically unavailable and cannot fulfill its role in bone-building and bone maintenance. Copper imbalances result from zinc and molybdenum deficiencies and environmental copper exposure via water pipes, copper cookware, birth-control pills, and dental materials. The Daily Reference Intake level for copper is 900 mcg for women 50 and older. The richest dietary sources are seafood, nuts, seeds, and organ meats such as liver.

MANGANESE

Your bones contain another mineral, manganese, that is involved in the production of enzymes needed to form collagen. Thus, this trace mineral is essential for synthesis of cartilage and other connective tissue, and for bone growth and maintenance. In a comparison of blood and bone samples of women with osteoporosis and women of the same age without osteoporosis, manganese levels were 75 percent lower in the women with the disease.

Manganese intake is cut in half when whole grains are replaced in our diets by refined flour. Foods high in phosphorus and calcium, as well as bran and other high-fiber foods, also tend to deplete manganese. To ensure that you are getting enough manganese in your diet, be sure to eat whole grains, nuts, seeds, sea vegetables, and dark leafy greens. Because this mineral is important to bone health and so many women do not get enough in their food because of poor dietary choices, you may also need to supplement food sources. The Daily Reference Intake level for women 50 and older is 1.8 mg. The best food sources of manganese are mainly vegetarian sources such as beans.

SILICON

High amounts of silicon have been found at calcification sites in growing bones. Silicon makes firm, strong tissues, promotes the formation of bones and teeth, and is a component of collagen. Plants contain silica, which human enzymes convert to silicon; theoretically, we should be able to get the silicon we need from vegetables and grains. However, food processing removes much of the silica, so most of us will need to use supplements, as I describe later. No Dietary Reference Intake value has been established for silicon. The best dietary sources are alfalfa; the hulls of wheat, oats, and rice; and the herbs nettle and horsetail.

ZINC

Our skeletons contain most of the zinc in our bodies. Three hundred different enzymes, many related to cell growth and health and our immune system, need zinc as a cofactor. Zinc is vital for normal bone formation and enhances the biochemical actions of vitamin D, which is vital in absorbing and transporting calcium. Unfortunately, as important as this mineral is, zinc deficiency is common in the United States. One dietary survey reported that 68 percent of adults in this country consume less than two-thirds the recommended level of zinc. In part, this is a result of food processing that removes zinc. In addition, twenty-two of the fifty states have soils that are deficient in zinc; foods grown in this soil are equally deficient. Finally, many of us avoid eating zinc-rich meat and eggs because of misguided cholesterol concerns (see Chapter 4) or unbalanced fad diets. The Daily Reference Intake level for zinc for women 50 and older is 8 mg. Good sources of zinc include eggs, meat, seafood (particularly oysters), pumpkin seeds, whole-grain cereals, dried beans, and legumes.

FOLIC ACID

Folic acid is an important vitamin factor in numerous health conditions. When it comes to bone issues, folic acid (also known as folate) may help prevent osteoporosis by lowering levels of the amino acid homocysteine. While high levels of homocysteine are primarily associated with the formation of atherosclerotic plaques (see Chapter 4), some evidence indicates too much homocysteine may also contribute to the development of osteoporosis by interfering with collagen formation. Folic acid, along with vitamins B_6 and B_{12}, converts the excess homocysteine into the antioxidant methionine and other chemicals that are used or excreted.

Like vitamin K, folic acid is produced by friendly intestinal bacteria. If you frequently take antibiotics, you may be susceptible to folic acid deficiency. Other common medications that deplete folic acid include aspirin, nonsteroidal anti-inflammatory drugs (NSAIDs), corticosteroids, anticonvulsants, and some cholesterol-lowering drugs. Excessive alcohol consumption and smoking block folic acid absorption, leading to a deficiency. The Daily Reference Intake value for folic acid is 400 mcg for women 50 and older. The best food sources are green leafy vegetables, tuna, salmon, cheese, brown rice, beef, beans, and barley.

VITAMIN B_6 (PYRIDOXINE)

Vitamin B_6 is a cofactor in more than a hundred enzyme reactions in the body, including production of lysyl oxidase, which strengthens connective tissue by cross-linking collagen strands. In conjunction with folic acid and vitamin B_{12}, vitamin B_6 also helps control levels of homocysteine to prevent its interference with collagen formation. Vitamin B_6 is produced by friendly intestinal bacteria. Amounts of the vitamin found in food are easily destroyed in cooking and food processing, so deficiencies are common. The Daily Reference Intake value for vitamin B_6 is 1.5 mg for women 50 and older. Among the best food sources are bananas, carrots, onions, asparagus, peas, sunflower seeds, walnuts, and wheat germ.

VITAMIN B_{12} (COBALAMIN)

The third B vitamin crucial to controlling homocysteine levels is vitamin B_{12}. It also enhances metabolism of the bone-building osteoblasts, thus aiding bone remodeling. Absorbed in the large intestine, vitamin

B_{12} is often deficient in older people, up to 30 percent of whom lack a chemical called "intrinsic factor" needed for the vitamin's absorption. A number of medications can cause a vitamin B_{12} deficiency, including antibiotics, antivirals, certain diabetes-control drugs, cholesterol-lowering medications, and ulcer drugs.

If you frequently experience gas and other digestive problems, be sure to chew your food well and consider supplementing daily with hydrochloric acid. The Daily Reference Intake value for vitamin B_{12} is 2.4 mcg for women 50 and older. Food sources include liver (beef and chicken), oysters, sardines, cheese, eggs, trout, salmon, and tuna. If you are vegetarian, you will have difficulty getting adequate vitamin B_{12} from your diet and may need to supplement.

VITAMIN C

Thanks to the work of Linus Pauling, Ph.D. (widely regarded as the Father of Vitamin C), and others, many of us are aware of the antioxidant and immune-boosting properties of vitamin C. We may be less aware of this vitamin's role in bone health. Vitamin C is essential in the formation of the structural protein collagen, an integral part of the body's connective tissue, bone, and teeth. Although probably one of the most well-known vitamins, vitamin C is deficient in the diet of many people, and up to 20 percent of those beyond the age of menopause are thought to be deficient.

The Daily Reference Intake value for vitamin C is 75 mg for women 50 and older; illness and all types of stress increase your need for the vitamin, so you may want to consider a supplement during menopause. However, a major Swedish study found that when women took high levels of both calcium and vitamin C, they had high rates of hip fractures, yet another reason to avoid taking too much calcium. When they reduced their intake of vitamin C, the fracture rate decreased. Our bodies cannot produce vitamin C, so food and supplements must provide what we need. The vitamin is destroyed by exposure to air, fluorescent light, and long-term storage, so there may be very little left by the time food sources reach our tables. Nevertheless, citrus fruits, cantaloupes, pineapples, strawberries, tomatoes, red and green peppers, cabbage, Brussels sprouts, and parsley are good sources of natural vitamin C.

VITAMIN D

Vitamin D ranks just behind calcium and magnesium in its importance to healthy bone formation. The body manufactures the vitamin from cholesterol when your skin is exposed to the ultraviolet rays of the sun. Vitamin D increases the absorption of both calcium and phosphorus from the intestine, helps release calcium from bone, and promotes calcium storage in the kidneys. At least one study has found that taking vitamin D supplements increased thighbone density by 2.7 percent in postmenopausal women. What you may not know is that recent research has linked vitamin D deficiencies to breast, prostate, colon, and skin cancers and to increased inflammation—which contributes to heart disease, arthritis, and diabetes—in otherwise healthy people.

Some experts estimate as many as 85 percent of Americans may be vitamin D deficient—particularly older people, for several reasons. First, their ability to transform vitamin D into its biologically active form, vitamin D_3, is impaired. Second, they may spend less time outdoors, getting less exposure to the sun. Finally, many medications deplete vitamin D, including certain antibiotics, cholesterol-lowering drugs, corticosteroids, and ulcer medications. The Daily Reference Intake level for vitamin D is 400 IU for women age 50 and older, but many experts, including Toronto researcher Reinhold Vieth, Ph.D., believe this level is inadequate. Pointing out that on a sunny summer day, we could produce 10,000 IU vitamin D if we were fully exposed, Vieth suggests that adults need at least 1000 to 2000 IU daily, primarily from supplements. In addition to adequate exposure to sunlight, sources of vitamin D include sardines, tuna, sweet potatoes and yams, alfalfa, and egg yolks.

VITAMIN K

Vitamin K is produced in your body by friendly intestinal bacteria. Although it is best known for its blood-clotting action, vitamin K is essential for the production of osteocalcin, a protein found only in bone and from which calcium is crystallized. When you lack osteocalcin, your bones become soft and weak. Vitamin K has also been shown to reduce the amount of calcium excreted in urine by as much as 50 percent in women with osteoporosis. Lower levels of vitamin K are associated with more severe osteoporotic fractures; the vitamin speeds the healing of fractures, apparently by stimulating bone growth. If you frequently take antibiotics, you may be particularly susceptible to a vitamin K deficiency, because the drugs destroy the bacteria needed to produce the vitamin. The Daily Reference Intake value for vitamin K is 90 mcg for women 50 and older. Dark green leafy vegetables, alfalfa, and kelp are rich sources of vitamin K; yogurt, egg yolks, and fish-liver oils are also good sources.

ESSENTIAL FATTY ACIDS

Essential fatty acids (EFAs) help make calcium available for tissue use and elevate calcium levels in your bloodstream. Unfortunately, because of our long history of fat phobia and penchant for processing foods, which destroys EFAs, most diets miss the boat on the powerhouses. Eating foods such as cold-water fish, seeds, nuts, and vegetable and botanical oils, which are rich in naturally occurring EFAs, can help correct this deficiency.

HYDROCHLORIC ACID: MISSING LINK TO CALCIUM ABSORPTION

Most of the calcium in foods and supplements is in the form of insoluble salts. These salts depend on an acidic stomach environment in order to dissolve and become bioavailable. Normally, the hydrochloric acid (HCl) in our stomachs creates the ideal acid pH, dissolving the calcium and breaking it down so it can be absorbed into the blood.

The acid in our stomachs also helps break down protein, as well as magnesium and other mineral cofactors to calcium metabolism. However, an estimated 40 percent of menopausal women are severely deficient in HCl, a condition known as achlorhydria. Studies by Robert Recker, M.D., and others have shown that people with low levels of HCl have poor calcium absorption.

Symptoms of achlorhydria include intestinal or stomach gas and bloating after meals. Age may be a factor, but so are drinking liquids with meals, chewing too little, or eating too fast. People with type A blood have a genetic predisposition to low levels of HCl. Unfortunately, when symptoms occur, many of us try over-the-counter antacids in the mistaken belief that the cause is too much acid. In fact, these antacids reduce the level of HCl even further, interfering with calcium absorption. This is true even for Tums, which is promoted as a source of calcium. Tums lacks calcium's major cofactor, magnesium, and reduces the very stomach acid needed to enhance the absorption of the calcium. A study of six thousand women, published in the *New England Journal of Medicine,* reported that women who used Tums as their only source of supplemental calcium had a higher rate of arm fractures than women who didn't. The reason for this may be that the calcium in Tums rarely gets out of the gut and into your body.

As we pass the age of 50, the chance we'll have inadequate levels of hydrochloric acid increases, so consider taking a hydrochloric acid supplement, especially if you have symptoms of gastric distress after eating. Look for one that includes pepsin, such as the formula from Country Life.

In addition to supplementing with HCl, you can enhance the acid pH in your stomach and thereby improve calcium absorption by eating foods high in calcium with small amounts of high-acid foods, such as lemon water, tomato juice, or vinegar. Chew your food well; signals from your taste buds stimulate HCl production. Avoid taking antacids and other acid-blocking drugs, unless you are under treatment for an ulcer, acid reflux disease, or other medical condition requiring lower acid levels.

Lifestyle

The health of your bones is a measure of the balance in your life, and not just in the calcium-magnesium or calcitonin-thyroxine ratios. Key lifestyle elements need to be in equilibrium as well. Like Goldilocks, you want them to be "not too hot, not too cold, but just right." Following are lifestyle practices that put you at risk for increased bone loss and osteoporosis.

EXCESSIVE USE OF ALCOHOL

It appears that alcohol suppresses the growth of new bone by poisoning bone-forming cells. In addition, alcohol has an extraordinarily negative effect on the ovaries, causing hormonal imbalances. Nutritional problems resulting from heavy alcohol use include irritation of the intestinal lining, leading to a decrease in absorption of nutrients, and liver damage, which interferes with the production of vitamin D, all of which will inevitably affect the development of strong bones.

SMOKING

Smoking more than doubles your risk of developing osteoporosis. Smokers often carry high levels of the toxic mineral cadmium in their blood, and one well-known result of high cadmium levels is a loss of calcium from bone, resulting in osteoporosis. Researchers also believe that smoking interferes with estrogen production and the way your body handles this hormone. Smokers have decreased blood and tissue levels of estrogen, and smoking leads to earlier menopause, leaving the body with lowered levels of estrogen for a longer period of time.

LACK OF EXERCISE

The familiar adage "use it or lose it" applies to bones. While the effect of weight-bearing exercise on muscle is obvious, its effect on your bones may be less obvious but is just as significant. Research has found that when muscles contract, the stress of the contraction is transmitted to the attached bone. This stress sets off an electrical charge that stimulates the osteoblasts to build bone. Bones are also strengthened when they bear weight—the weight of your moving body, strength balls, free weights, or machine weights. Postmenopausal women who carry out regular weight-bearing exercise can see an average 6 percent increase in bone density of their lower spine by the end of one year. Regular exercise also appears to protect against hip fractures, lowering the risk for those of us who exercise to half that of women who are sedentary.

Weight-bearing exercise is the best physical activity for increasing bone mass. Regular exercise via brisk walking, jogging, dancing, playing tennis or other racquet sports, jumping rope, and strength training (with hand weights, bands, or weighted balls) is good for preserving bone—if you do at least 90 minutes a week. Swimming, cycling, yoga, and stretching put only minimal stress on the body, so these exercises, while healthful, do not enhance your bone health. You can read more about my Hot Times Exercise Prescription in Chapter 6.

Balance is the key, however, for too much strenuous or vigorous exercise can have a negative effect: It lowers body fat levels to the point that estrogen production is slowed, thereby affecting calcium absorption. Lowered body fat is also tied to irregularities in menstruation. I've consistently noted that body fat must be maintained at a minimum of about 18 percent for women to continue a normal menstrual cycle. Any condition that interferes with the menstrual cycle can lower bone density.

STAYING TOO THIN

Like exercise-induced weight loss, continual, prolonged, or on-again-off-again dieting habits can severely interfere with hormonal and calcium function. Obsession with weight and dieting leads too many women to resort to extremely low-calorie diets that lack sufficient amounts of calcium and other bone-building elements. This inadequate consumption, coupled with absorption problems, triggers your body to pull more calcium from your bones to stabilize falling blood levels. Thin women are more at risk of osteoporosis for many reasons: They have less bone mass to start with; they do not absorb as much calcium because they lack estrogen-producing fat (which in turn leads to bone loss); and they benefit less from the metabolic bone-building function of fat on bone.

My approach to osteoporosis is, like the disease itself, multifaceted. We need to be aware of all the factors contributing to our risk of this disease and work toward changing those factors over which we have control. We do have a choice in how our bodies age. We can make positive lifestyle and dietary choices that can slow down and eliminate many of the risks of developing this degenerative disease. By improving and supplementing our diets to aid in proper absorption of nutrients, by eliminating unhealthy lifestyle habits, and by participating in regular weight-bearing exercise, we can improve and support our bones. The choice is ours.

FOUR

Heart Disease

An Important Note About Heart Disease
Please read this chapter, even if heart disease "doesn't run in your family," even if you have low cholesterol levels and your blood pressure is normal, even if you believe you should be more concerned about breast cancer than heart disease. Despite what you may think, the next few pages may be among the most important you will read today because there's so much "new news" about heart disease as it relates to women. The guidelines in this chapter can be used for both prevention and treatment.

FOR VARIOUS REASONS, HEART DISEASE HAS TRADITIONALLY been thought of as a man's disease. Unfortunately, this view has affected the way physicians have dealt with their female patients, the way research has been conducted, and the way women have sought care. Until recently, almost all we knew about heart disease and its treatment related to men. One reason for this is that women develop the problem about ten years later than men do. Another reason is that women were excluded from most of the major studies on heart disease prior to the early 1990s. The early studies that did use women subjects were conducted for shorter periods of time with smaller numbers of subjects and provided less data and no long-term results. These factors, plus some others I will discuss shortly, led to heart disease being ignored or undiagnosed in women, and being far more advanced by the time women sought or received medical care. Even those who sought care early were often not taken seriously. In fact, studies have found that women's chest pains are more likely to be diagnosed as psychiatric than men's are.

Fortunately, this picture is changing, if slowly. A closer look at the statistics reveals some startling and sobering facts:

- One in three women will develop cardiovascular disease, including heart disease, high blood pressure (hypertension), or stroke, during her lifetime.
- A half million American women will die this year from cardiovascular disease, which is the leading cause of death in women.
- Heart attacks alone kill six times as many women each year as breast cancer.

What Causes Heart Disease?

Simply put, cardiovascular disease results when the lumens of the coronary arteries, which carry blood, oxygen, and nutrients to the heart, become smaller. This constriction can be caused by excess salt in the blood pulling fluid from the arteries. Arteries are further constricted by a buildup of fats, oxidized cholesterol, excess calcium, and plaque in the artery walls. Angina, or chest pain, occurs when the heart fails to receive enough oxygen through these narrowed arteries. When these arteries become obstructed, a heart attack can occur, resulting in damage to the heart tissue. This process of plaque buildup and obstruction is known as atherosclerosis, or hardening of the arteries.

As a result of recent major studies, we now know that the pattern heart disease follows in women is notably different from the pattern it follows in men. First, although heart disease can occur at any age, in women it becomes a significant health factor during menopause—about ten years later than in men.

Second, women are less likely to experience the classic crushing chest pain many men describe. A woman's symptoms are much more subtle, often starting weeks or even months before an attack. Women may describe "not feeling quite right," with symptoms such as shortness of breath, unusual weakness or fatigue, sleep disturbances, chest discomfort that may come and go quickly, vision problems, anxiety, and indigestion. The vagueness of these symptoms leads women to ignore them, delaying treatment. When these women do seek treatment, their doctor may misdiagnose their condition.

Third, the disease itself develops differently in women. According to researchers at the University of Michigan Cardiovascular Center, significant blockages tend to occur not in major arteries but in smaller, less flexible blood vessels. When diagnostic coronary angiography is performed, the major vessels appear clear. This helps account for some of the differences in treatment women receive, conclude the Michigan researchers. Coronary angioplasty, a procedure to clear blockages, and coronary bypass surgery are both better suited to larger blood vessels.

All these factors may help account for the dismal prognosis for women with heart disease. Women who have heart attacks do not seem to recover as quickly or as fully as men, and nearly 40 percent of women die within the first year after their first diagnosed attack.

Women are twice as likely as men to die after bypass surgery. A study from the Mayo Clinic Women's Heart Clinic found 57 percent of women suffered depression or anxiety from their heart disease, which may explain why only about 1 in 10 women makes lifestyle changes after a heart attack.

If these circumstances are to change, we need to be more aggressive in seeking a diagnosis and treatment and in making lifestyle changes. Mayo Clinic cardiologist Sharonne Hayes suggests we need to be evaluated differently from men. We should take not only a stress (or treadmill) test, which records the heart's electrical activity during exercise, but also a nuclear scan (also known as a thallium stress test) or an EKG. Another diagnostic tool more recently developed is electron-beam computed tomography, which is a quick, noninvasive scan that detects calcium deposits in the lining of arteries. It is particularly effective in diagnosing early heart disease, although you may have to travel to a major cardiac center to have the test performed. Perhaps most important, all of us need to evaluate our risk of heart disease and take steps to change our lifestyle to lower as many of those risks as possible.

UNDERSTANDING YOUR
RISK FACTORS

To date, at least 250 risk factors for heart disease have been identified. You'll be glad to know many of these risk factors, especially those with the greatest impact on risk, can be lowered by lifestyle changes such as those in the Hot Times approach. However, two risk factors associated with heart disease are beyond your control: heredity and age. For both men and women, the closer your blood tie to a relative who suffered from heart disease, the greater your risk of developing it. In addition, age is a factor for women. As you reach menopause, your risk of developing heart disease rises significantly. Of the estimated 435,000 American women who have heart attacks each year, 426,000 are age 45 or older.

We can't choose the families we're born into, and few of us would choose a shorter life to lower our risk of a heart attack. What we can do is choose to live a healthier lifestyle that could lower many of the other risk factors. Let's look more closely at some of the most important factors, starting with the best-known and moving to some of the most recently discovered.

High Blood Pressure

Hypertension, or high blood pressure, is both a cause and an effect of cardiovascular disease. The exact cause of hypertension is generally unknown, but what we do know is that high blood pressure often accompanies heart disease. The excessive force of the blood against the arteries weakens the cellular walls, allowing LDL ("bad") cholesterol, excess calcium, and other toxic substances to form deposits that eventually block the arteries. Almost 50 percent of all midlife women are diagnosed with hypertension by age 50. Most who have hypertension are unaware of it because it usually produces no physical symptoms. Routine blood pressure checks, at least every two years, can detect potential hypertension; blood pressure readings above 140/90 may spell danger.

Because so many test results have shown a direct relationship between high salt intake and hypertension, removing the salt shaker from your table would be wise. Sodium is a factor in hypertension because it causes fluid retention, which adds stress to both the heart and the circulatory system. Hypertension, left undiagnosed or untreated, can result in stroke, heart attack, kidney failure, and other serious diseases. Nearly 30 percent of the adult white population and over one-third of the adult black population suffer from high blood pressure.

Smoking

Let's face facts: if you smoke, your chances of dying from heart disease are almost three times as great as those of dying from lung cancer. The negative effects of smoking on your cardiovascular system are related to several actions. Nicotine causes blood platelets to become sticky, increasing plaque formation. Smoking also has been shown to decrease levels of HDL ("good") cholesterol and increase LDL ("bad") cholesterol. Cigarettes are high in cadmium, a toxic mineral that damages heart tissue.

The Nurses' Health Study, conducted by Harvard researchers, found that women who smoked just one to four cigarettes a day had nearly two and one-half times the rate of heart disease of nonsmokers. Keep in mind that even secondhand smoke increases your risk of heart disease, so make your home and car smoke-free environments.

Obesity

Unfortunately for us, weight appears to be a more significant risk factor for women than it is for men. A study by Harvard researcher JoAnn Manson, M.D., found that in obese women, seven out of ten cases of heart disease resulted from their excess weight. Even women who are at the high end of their "normal" range seem to have an increased risk. To compound the problem, overweight women tend to be sedentary; they are also more likely to develop hypertension, high LDL cholesterol and triglycerides, and type 2 diabetes, all of which increase the likelihood of heart disease.

How the weight is distributed on your body also seems to have an impact. Women with an apple body shape—who have a proportionally higher amount of fat around their abdomen than elsewhere on their body—have higher rates of heart disease, hypertension, and diabetes than their pear-shaped sisters, who carry their excess fat in their hips and thighs. Scientists believe this association relates to the hormone cortisol, which causes fatty acids to be released into the bloodstream from the central fat cells. These cells are located close to your liver; the released fatty acids stress the liver, causing cholesterol, blood pressure, and insulin levels to rise. Psychology researcher Elissa S. Epel has also discovered that apple-shaped women feel stress more and produce more cortisol as a result than do pear-shaped women.

Diabetes

For us women, diabetes is an additional risk factor for heart disease. Blood platelets in diabetics seem to stick together more readily than in nondiabetics, causing clogging of the arteries. Diabetics also have higher total cholesterol and lower HDL cholesterol levels. Research shows that women over the age of 45 are twice as likely as men to develop type 2 (formerly known as adult-onset) diabetes, and female diabetics are at double the risk of heart disease of male diabetics. The good news is that type 2 diabetes can be managed with diet and exercise, a subject covered more extensively in the next chapter.

A Sedentary Lifestyle

Movies depicting life on the nineteenth-century American frontier and Canadian wilderness are harsh reminders of just how physically demanding everyday life once was. We might enjoy watching someone else chop wood, carry buckets of water long distances, and walk behind a plowhorse, but few of us would trade in our computers, microwave ovens, and central heating to live that life.

All our muscles, including our heart, need exercise, however. Exercise helps lower LDL cholesterol and raise HDL cholesterol. Regular aerobic exercise—such as walking, running, jumping rope, and dancing—reduces the risk of heart disease by about 30 percent in postmenopausal women. It also influences several other risk factors. People who exercise regularly have a 35 percent lower risk of hyper-

tension, as well as a lower risk of diabetes. Exercise stimulates production of serotonin, endorphins, and other brain chemicals that reduce anxiety and stress and create a balanced sleep-wake cycle,
helping to control cortisol levels. When you exercise, you also aid
calcium metabolism, triggering the calcification process within your
bones so excess calcium does not build up in your blood vessels.

And you don't even need to spend one to two hours a day in strenuous activity to achieve cardiovascular benefits. As I discuss in greater
detail in Chapter 6, overexercising can be just as harmful as being a
couch potato. Moderate exercise, performed regularly, such as with
my Hot Times Exercise Prescription, significantly decreases your risk
of heart disease.

Cholesterol Levels

Almost all of us are aware of the connection between cholesterol and
heart disease. We know that cholesterol is carried through the bloodstream in two forms, HDL and LDL. The HDL is considered the
"good" cholesterol, and the LDL the "bad." An excess of LDL increases our risk of heart attacks and strokes, while high levels of
HDL protect us. In general, total cholesterol levels higher than 200
mg/dL can be a sign of increased risk for heart disease. In women,
LDL levels should be below 130 mg/dL and optimum HDL levels
should be greater than 50 mg/dL. More important than just these
single levels, however, the ratio of total cholesterol to HDL should be
below 4:1.

But in all the press coverage of cholesterol, some basic facts are
usually ignored. Cholesterol is found naturally in every cell in our
body, and each cell also contains enzymes used for the production of
cholesterol. Our brains and spinal cord have about 25 percent of our
bodies' stores of cholesterol. This important substance is found in the
skin, where it is converted to vitamin D by sunlight; in the marrow of

our bones, where blood cells are formed; and in our adrenal glands, where it is used in the formation of sex hormones, especially those found in postmenopausal women. Cholesterol is essential to good health, and deficiencies have been associated with anemia, acute infection, and excess thyroid function. In our diets, cholesterol is the waxy fatlike substance found only in products of animal origin, such as beef, poultry, and eggs.

So if cholesterol is so vitally important to our health, why have we been led to believe we need to avoid it in our diets? The concern over dietary cholesterol began with a 1913 Russian study by Nikolai Anitschkov, a physiologist. He found that feeding rabbits huge doses of cholesterol caused a dramatic rise in cholesterol in their blood. The resulting hardening of the arteries was blamed on cholesterol, because it was found at the site of arterial damage. From this, the theory developed that diets high in cholesterol caused heart disease, and an advertising campaign was launched promoting the idea that processed substitutes for dairy items, eggs, and butter are healthier for us than the natural foods on which they are based.

There's no denying a relationship exists between high dietary cholesterol levels and high levels in blood, but it's not as straightforward as we've been led to believe. How do we explain patients whose blood cholesterol levels are no lower after eating a very low-fat diet? How do we explain a much lower rate of second heart attacks in patients on a typical high-cholesterol diet over patients on a restricted diet?

What the research seems to suggest is the amount of cholesterol in one's blood is related to heart disease, while the amount of cholesterol in one's diet is not. *What does lead to high blood cholesterol is the lack of other nutrients—such as chromium, magnesium, vitamin B_3, and omega-3 essential fatty acids—needed to metabolize cholesterol.* In addition, cholesterol accumulates in arteries only after the arterial wall has been damaged. Cholesterol, in and of itself, is not the villain it has been made out to be. In fact, 50 percent of Americans who have heart attacks have levels of total cholesterol that are normal or only moderately elevated.

Pure, fresh cholesterol does not damage arteries, but oxygenated cholesterol does. Cholesterol that has been exposed to oxygen produces toxic substances that decompose into free radicals, a term that has become synonymous with cell and tissue destruction. Free radicals are present in cholesterol that has oxidized as a result of exposure to air, high temperatures, free radical initiators, light, or a combination of these factors. They are unstable and highly reactive oxygen molecules with unpaired electrons, and they search for and steal electrons from other molecules, causing a chemical reaction that creates even more free radicals. It is free radicals that cause the damage to our blood vessel walls. Free radicals also cause other damage within cells by attacking membranes, proteins, and DNA. Reexamination of the Anitschkov and other animal feeding studies have found that the cholesterol used was not in the form in which it occurs naturally in food, but as heat-dried egg-yolk powder made up in batches to last many days or weeks. This altered cholesterol, because of its exposure to oxygen, formed free radicals.

Oxidized cholesterol from food sources that are left out at room temperature or are fired, smoked, cured (sausage), or aged (cheese) can be highly plaque-producing. Cholesterol in our diets is dangerous only when it becomes oxidized, and processing, packaging, storage, and preparing of foods have a profound effect on oxidation. Animal foods cause problems when they have been exposed to the ravages of oxygen for extended periods of time—for example, improperly stored eggs, milk, or butter that is exposed to room temperature for long periods of time or not stored in tightly sealed containers. Other sources of oxidized cholesterol can be found in many fast foods—fried chicken, fried fish, and hamburgers. Dried milk, dried eggs, and packaged dry baking mixes (for custards, cakes, puddings, pancakes) are also on the list. These are some of the greatest sources of oxidized cholesterol, and they are the very products often touted and recommended for their cholesterol-lowering effects!

Again, I'm not saying that diets high in fats and cholesterol are not related to heart disease, but the relationship is different from what we have been led to believe. Fats and cholesterol don't just clog up arteries. They are a major source of those nasty molecules the free radicals, which oxidize cells and set off a chain reaction, creating more and more free radicals. To make matters worse, the cholesterol manufactured by our bodies to fight against the damage done by free radicals is converted into its oxidized form. This only leads to more free radicals.

So how do we stop this chain reaction? We need to prevent the oxidation of cholesterol. By avoiding foods that contain oxidized cholesterol and damaged fats and increasing your intake of foods rich in antioxidant vitamins, minerals, and essential fatty acids (EFAs), you can decrease your risk of heart disease. Antioxidants are nutrients capable of neutralizing those nasty free radicals. Your body doesn't produce antioxidants, so you must get them from diet and supplementation. More and more research shows heart disease is related to deficiencies of these nutrients, including vitamins E, C, and A and the minerals selenium, chromium, zinc, and magnesium. The Hot Times approach to heart disease, outlined later in this chapter, ensures you get these vital nutrients every day.

Heart-healthy diets—those that are low in fat and cholesterol and designed to lower serum cholesterol levels—are a standard recommendation for anyone with elevated cholesterol. Yet in the two decades since the U.S. National Institutes of Health officially recommended the low-fat diet, obesity and type 2 diabetes rates have soared and heart disease rates have remained unchanged. Low-fat diets are particularly questionable for women, in whom levels of "good" (HDL) cholesterol are key in the prevention of heart disease. When men go on some special diets, such as one endorsed by the American Heart Association, they are able to reduce their LDL levels without affect-

ing their HDL levels. But in women, this same diet results in reduction of both LDL and HDL. In men, the risk of heart disease seems
to be primarily affected by a rise in LDL levels. For us, however, lowering HDL levels may increase our risk of heart disease even if LDL
levels are lowered at the same time.

Women should keep in mind that HDL levels above 50 mg/dL are
now considered the most desirable; levels between 40 and 50 indicate borderline risk of heart disease. "Bad" (LDL) cholesterol levels
should optimally be less than 130. Levels between 130 and 159 suggest borderline risk, while levels greater than 159 indicate high risk.
A low-fat diet is not the best way for a woman to maintain these levels. But the Hot Times Diet's increased fiber intake (especially in the
form of flaxseed oil) and cholesterol-lowering supplements can help
women lower LDL levels and increase their intake of antioxidants.

Fiber in the form of ground flaxseed, oat bran, and psyllium husks
has proved effective in lowering LDL and raising HDL, and can be
used in tasty oat bran muffins and cleansing drinks. The old stand-
bys, garlic and olive oil, are two other foods that seem to be beneficial
to women's cholesterol levels. The omega-3 fatty acids found in fish
oils, fish, and vegetable oils such as flaxseed oil are heart-smart
because they dramatically reduce both cholesterol and triglycerides
without affecting the beneficial HDLs. Another attractive benefit is
their ability to lower blood pressure. Flaxseed oil is a buttery, nutty-
tasting oil that makes a good butter substitute. It can be drizzled over
steamed vegetables, cooked cereals, and air-popped popcorn for a
rich, satisfying flavor. It makes a good base for salad dressings, such
as my Cranberry Lover's Salad Dressing (page 227). Flaxseed oil
should not be used for cooking, as heat destroys its value.

Luckily, there are a number of easy-to-take nutrients that can help
us lower our cholesterol safely. Both chromium and vitamin C have
been shown to lower plasma cholesterol while increasing HDL levels. Chromium is well known for its role in cholesterol metabolism
and protects the lining of the arteries from damage, thereby prevent-

ing buildup of cholesterol in the arteries. Vitamin C appears to prevent LDL oxidation.

Vitamin E has long been known as a potent antioxidant. It has been shown to scavenge free radicals and increase internal antioxidation. Vitamin E also helps thin the blood. It inhibits blood platelets from becoming sticky, thereby reducing blood-clotting problems. This is especially beneficial for women, who do not seem to be able to tolerate the one-a-day blood-thinning aspirin routine. Vitamin E is also protective of two other antioxidant vitamins, A and C. When E is present, less A and C is required. (For my specific recommendations, see page 22.)

Triglycerides

Although triglycerides are another type of blood fat, the important relationship they have to women and heart disease warrants a special mention. As I discuss above, high triglyceride levels are known to increase a woman's susceptibility to heart disease even when cholesterol levels are normal. While many experts say that triglyceride levels above 150 mg/dL are cause for concern, I believe you need to closely monitor levels above 100.

Your liver makes triglycerides from refined sugars, and you get additional triglycerides from the fats and oils you eat. In your bloodstream, sticky triglyceride particles act like glue, causing red blood cells to clump and stick together. Your small capillaries become blocked, leading to oxygen starvation of the tissues and organs served by these capillaries. Triglycerides are also the form in which the body stores fat in the connective tissue. The roll above many a middle-aged stomach is actually caused by excess triglycerides.

What we eat and the way we live affect our triglyceride levels. The low-fat, high-carbohydrate diet encouraged by the American Heart Association, the USDA, and others actually raises triglyceride levels and lowers HDL levels in up to one-third of Americans. White sugar, white flour, and products such as white bread, cakes, cookies, candies, soda, and alcohol all increase our triglycerides. Even too much fruit and natural, unsweetened fruit juice can elevate levels. Eating fat can double blood triglycerides, but drinking some beer with your burger can increase the levels three and a half times. A few drinks before a fatty meal that is followed by a sugary dessert can truly spell disaster.

Not only what we eat, but the *way* we eat affects our triglyceride levels. If you skip breakfast and/or lunch and make up for it with a heavy evening meal (sound familiar?), you boost your blood triglycerides. Eating a large meal late in the day causes your body to store unused triglycerides in fatty tissue; skipping breakfast the next day results in those triglycerides flooding out of the fatty tissue and sludging up the bloodstream. Our bodies were designed to be fueled at regular intervals with good, balanced food. If we're not eating regularly, we're damaging our bodies.

Other behaviors that contribute to high triglyceride levels include lack of physical activity, reaction to emotional stress, and consumption of caffeine, nicotine, certain drugs such as diuretics and birth control pills, and some hormones, including estrogen. Both triglyceride and cholesterol levels increase naturally with age, so have them checked every couple of years as a routine part of your health care.

Trans Fats

Within the past hundred years, the rate of cardiovascular disease has risen 350 percent, but the cholesterol content of the American diet has remained about the same. During this same hundred years, however, both sugar and processed oil consumption have risen considerably. Hydrogenated polyunsaturated oils, including margarine, have been recommended for years in cholesterol-lowering diets, and while it is true that these oils will reduce cholesterol levels, it is also true that they accelerate arteriosclerosis and other degenerative diseases.

Why? Because oils that have been commercially processed to improve shelf life, flavor, smell, and color have been damaged. In the processing, high temperatures convert the polyunsaturated fatty acids from the naturally occurring beneficial "cis" to the unnatural, harmful "trans" form. Cis fats melt at 55°F, well below the normal body temperature of 98.6°F, which makes them fully available to the system. Trans fats melt at up to 111°F, so they remain solid, and therefore unmetabolized, in the human body.

The process of hydrogenation, which converts liquid oils into hardened fats such as margarine and vegetable shortening, destroys natural fatty acids in even greater numbers, converting them into the biologically impaired trans form. Trans fats, found in all processed oils on your grocery shelves and in margarines (which have the highest percentage of trans-fatty acids), cannot be used by the body to produce prostaglandins, hormone-like compounds that regulate every function in the human body at the molecular level. These trans fats interfere with normal cell membrane function and structure, and block the good healthy fats, such as raw natural oils that make prostaglandins, from being taken in. In addition to these trans fats, the hydrogenation process also removes the very nutrients that are essential for healthy hearts—vitamins E and B_6, chromium, and magnesium.

C-Reactive Protein Levels

In his book *Heart Sense for Women*, cardiologist Stephen Sinatra identifies a number of risk factors for heart disease that have only very recently been explored—factors he calls "new millennium risk factors." Among them is C-reactive protein (CRP), which could be more important than cholesterol in identifying a woman's risk of heart disease.

C-reactive protein is a natural chemical, produced in the liver in response to chronic or acute inflammation. What researchers now know is that atherosclerosis is an inflammatory disease that sets off your body's immune response. Whether plaque builds up on the inside of your arteries, causing blockages, or grows into the vessel walls, causing them to bulge outward, the immune response sends thousands of special cells to attack the plaque. At the same time, your liver produces CRP to help rid your body of the plaque. Unfortunately, this process destabilizes the plaque, which can break apart and cause blood clots that can lead to heart attack or stroke. In addition, researchers at the University of California–Davis have discovered that CRP can stimulate production of an enzyme known to block clot breakdown; CRP has even been identified as the cause of artery inflammation and plaque buildup in some people.

Paul Ridker, M.D., and his colleagues at Brigham and Women's Hospital in Boston have carried out some of the most extensive research to date on CRP and heart disease in women. Following 28,000 women for eight years, his group found that women who had high CRP levels and low LDL cholesterol had a greater risk of heart attack than women who had low CRP levels and high LDL, making CRP a stronger predictor of heart attack and stroke. Based on results from more than a dozen studies, people with the highest levels of CRP have twice the risk of heart attacks compared with those having the lowest levels.

Levels of CRP may explain why low-cholesterol diets fail to prevent heart disease in some people. Researchers at Johns Hopkins found that healthy middle-aged people who followed a low-cholesterol diet had a greater rise in their triglyceride levels and a smaller decrease in their blood cholesterol levels if they had high CRP levels.

We don't yet know if lowering CRP levels can lower your incidence of heart attack and stroke. While we wait for the research results, you may want to ask your doctor about having your CRP levels measured. A simple blood test is all that is needed, and it is often performed as part of an entire lipid screen. In 2003, the American Heart Association and Centers for Disease Control and Prevention published guidelines to help you and your doctor in evaluating the need for the test and its results. The recommendation is that people with an "intermediate risk" of heart disease have their CRP levels measured. That includes people with a few of the risk factors I've just discussed, which gives them a 10 to 20 percent chance of developing heart disease within ten years—an estimated 40 percent of the adult U.S. population, or about 100 million men and women, fall into this intermediate risk category. Because CRP is released in response to any inflammation, people who have arthritis, lupus, and other autoimmune disorders or who have recently experienced acute illness or injury will not get accurate results with regard to their risk of heart disease. Medications including corticosteroids, cholesterol-lowering drugs (statins), and NSAIDs lower CRP levels, giving an inaccurate picture of your heart risk. A test result of 3 mg/l or more indicates a high risk and is a signal to take steps to lower your CRP, including losing weight if you are overweight; getting regular aerobic exercise; stopping smoking; consuming a diet low in saturated and trans fat and high in vitamin D, such as the Hot Times Diet, described in Chapter 7; and reducing stress.

Magnesium Deficiency

Just as the role of magnesium, boron, and the other essential vitamins and trace minerals in the prevention of osteoporosis has been overshadowed by the focus on calcium, the role of magnesium in protection against heart disease has been virtually ignored because of the cholesterol craze and emphasis on estrogen. We all know that high cholesterol levels are somehow related to heart disease, but most of us are unaware that magnesium deficiencies can result in heart conditions such as irregular heartbeat and rapid heartbeat, high blood pressure, and sudden death. Magnesium deficiency may also be the cause of idiopathic mitral valve prolapse, a heart valve disorder whose symptoms include palpitations, chest pain, fatigue, panic attacks, and hyperventilation. Low levels of both blood and cellular magnesium have been reported in individuals with high blood pressure and hypertension, and biopsies reveal that individuals who die from heart attacks have lower magnesium levels in their heart muscle than those who died of other causes.

To add to the problem, many people with high blood pressure are prescribed diuretics or fluid pills to treat swelling and fluid retention that actually *cause* both magnesium and potassium deficiencies, which can exacerbate their heart condition. The powerful cardiac drug digitalis also affects how well your body uses both magnesium and potassium. Often, potassium is prescribed along with digitalis, but magnesium is neglected. This is unsound nutritional medicine, because the body requires magnesium in order to use potassium. Drugs used to treat arrhythmia (irregular heartbeat), such as quinidine sulfate and disopyramide phosphate, are also known to induce a magnesium deficiency. In order to avoid all of these heart health complications, magnesium supplementation, in addition to the generally prescribed potassium, should be part of every nutritional protocol for women taking cardiac drugs.

Magnesium deficiencies can actually hasten the development of atherosclerosis, or hardening of the arteries. If you have a calcium-magnesium imbalance, calcium doesn't become part of the bone as it should. This unused calcium then gets dumped into the arteries and becomes part of the "hardened" artery. With the food industry pumping supplemental calcium into every possible food and beverage, many of us surely have excess calcium, out of balance with magnesium and other minerals, deposited in our arteries. We must bring magnesium levels back into balance with calcium to keep this excess calcium out of our blood vessels.

Instead of assessing magnesium levels and increasing this important mineral to its proper ratio with calcium, the doctors of many heart patients with potential magnesium deficiencies prescribe calcium channel blockers. Procardia, Cardizem, Cardene, and Isoptin or Calan are used to prevent heart muscle spasms by blocking excess calcium from being absorbed into the heart muscle. Magnesium is a natural calcium channel blocker; it dilates coronary arteries and peripheral arteries when available in sufficient levels and in balance with calcium, yet it is overlooked as a key factor in maintaining a healthy heart.

Magnesium is not just essential for bone health and osteoporosis prevention; it is equally vital to muscle health and in the prevention and treatment of heart disease. Calcium helps make muscles contract, but magnesium helps them relax. For the heart this is crucial, because if it is under constant stress, it cannot function properly. Hard drinking water, which is high in magnesium and calcium content, has been linked to low rates of serious heart disease. In fact, intravenous magnesium has been successfully used for over fifty years in the treatment of coronary spasms and heart attacks.

Sufficient magnesium also has been shown to lower total cholesterol, LDL cholesterol, and triglyceride levels while raising HDL cholesterol. This is especially good news for us, because diets designed to lower LDL levels often lower HDL levels as well, which in women leads to an increased risk of heart disease. Magnesium also reduces platelet aggregation, the stickiness of blood cells, which contributes to their clumping in your arteries.

A USDA nationwide food consumption survey found that the typical American diet provides about two-thirds of the recommended 320 mg of magnesium a day. Some experts recommend up to 800 to 1000 mg of magnesium. The depletion of our soil and the overprocessing and overcooking of our food rob it of much of its magnesium content. Excesses in sugar, alcohol, fiber, caffeine, "bad" fats, and phosphates in sodas and other processed foods sap our bodies of magnesium, as does that ever-present twentieth-century condition: stress. Table 4-1 (page 116) lists foods that are high in magnesium. I also suggest supplementing with an additional 400 mg of magnesium alone or taking it in a multiple supplement such as Uni Key's Female Multiple.

Table 4-1 Foods High in Magnesium

Food	Mg/100 g edible portion*
Kelp	760
Wheat bran	490
Wheat germ	336
Almonds	270
Cashews	267
Blackstrap molasses	258
Brewer's yeast	231
Buckwheat	229
Brazil nut	225
Dulse	220
Filberts	184
Peanuts	175
Millet	162
Wheat grain	160
Pecan	142
English walnut	131
Rye	115
Tofu	111
Coconut meat, dry	90
Soybeans, cooked	88
Spinach (raw)	88
Brown rice	88
Dried figs	71
Swiss chard	65
Apricots, dried (unsulfured)	62
Dates	58
Collard greens	57
Shrimp	51
Sweet corn	48
Avocado	45
Cheddar cheese	45
Parsley	41
Prunes, dried	40

Data from Endo-met Laboratories, Phoenix, Arizona, based on evaluation of existing literature.

*100 g = 3.5 oz.

The traditional blood test to measure magnesium is considered useless in assessing magnesium deficiency, because the body tries to maintain a balance of magnesium in the blood at all times. When blood levels drop, magnesium is pulled from other parts of the body, so blood tests generally show adequate levels of magnesium when in reality you may be severely deficient. One of the most accurate diagnostic tests available at the present is called the magnesium loading test, which tests urine rather than blood. You might want to ask your doctor about it.

Homocysteine Levels

Thirty-five years ago, Kilmer McCully, M.D., proposed homocysteine as a factor in damage to blood vessels and heart disease, but it has only been within the past five to ten years that substantial research results have overcome medical skepticism. Researchers are still trying to identify the exact role of homocysteine in not only heart disease but also rheumatoid arthritis, diabetes, and possibly osteoporosis.

Here's what we know at present: Methionine is an amino acid present in red meat, poultry, legumes, eggs, avocado, and grains that helps prevent cholesterol from clogging your arteries. During methionine metabolism, homocysteine (another amino acid) is formed. Under ideal circumstances, the homocysteine is broken down into other chemicals and used or eventually excreted. If conditions are less than ideal, however, blood homocysteine levels rise, damaging cell membranes, destabilizing collagen, and paving the way for cholesterol to form plaques. Among the factors known to increase homocysteine levels are:

- deficiencies in vitamins B_6 and B_{12} and folic acid (folate)
- smoking
- excessive coffee consumption (eight cups a day or more)

- taking anticonvulsant, antibacterial, diuretic, and some chemotherapy medications
- having kidney failure or hypothyroidism (see the next chapter)

Most recently, researchers have identified a genetic enzyme defect
that leads to high homocysteine levels, a defect present in an estimated 5 percent of the population.

If you are a woman with high blood pressure and high homocysteine levels, you have 25 times the risk of having a heart attack or
stroke than women with normal readings of both. Just how valuable
homocysteine results are in evaluating heart disease risk in healthy
women is still being studied. In the meantime, follow the Hot Times
approach to heart disease to be sure you're getting the vitamins you
need. Talk with your doctor about evaluating your homocysteine levels with either of two blood tests currently available.

Ferritin Levels

With menopause comes the cessation of menstruation, and some researchers have been looking into a possible connection between the
increased risk of coronary disease and declining blood loss. It appears
that at least one connection may be the accumulation of iron.

Iron is an essential mineral for blood production, absorption of
cadmium, production of key enzymes, and protection against aluminum absorption. Unlike other minerals, however, excess iron is
not excreted, but is stored in tissues, accumulating indefinitely. In
particular, women age 55 to 65 experience a doubling of the level
of ferritin, a protein-carrying iron. Ferritin, like C-reactive protein,
also increases in the presence of inflammation. During menstruation,
women lose iron, so the levels of ferritin circulating in blood are kept
under control. Without this natural release, however, iron accumulates and iron overload can occur, causing hair loss, fatigue, abdominal pain, irritable bowel syndrome, and heart disease. When excess

iron is stored in heart tissue, it contributes to heart muscle damage. Some researchers believe that when the ferritin iron is released from its protein, free radicals are formed that oxidize cholesterol. As I've described, this oxidized cholesterol clings to artery walls, forming plaques that can block the artery, leading to heart attack and stroke.

About 10 percent of the population has a genetic predisposition to iron overload, making them particularly vulnerable to its effects on the heart. At least one study has found that for every 1 percent increase in ferritin levels, the risk of heart disease rises 4 percent. Ask your doctor about a serum ferritin test to determine your own iron level. Avoid taking iron supplements once you have stopped menstruating and moderate your intake of iron-rich foods, such as red meat, spinach, and iron-fortified grains.

A Few Words About Estrogen and Heart Disease

Heart disease is one of the many conditions associated with menopause that physicians have routinely treated with estrogen replacement therapy (ERT) or hormone replacement therapy (HRT). The treatment was based partly on assumptions that reduced levels of estrogen were a cause of heart disease. Some studies seem to support this assumption, but a number of others do not. While estrogen use seems to reduce LDL cholesterol and increase HDL cholesterol, it also increases triglyceride levels, a known risk factor for heart attack. Estrogen also has the potential to raise blood pressure and increase blood clotting, leading to stroke.

In fact, in 2002, the U.S. Women's Health Initiative study of two forms of HRT was halted early because of an increased risk of heart disease and blood clots among women taking Prempro. (For more on the effects of HRT, see Chapter 1.) The National Heart,

Lung, and Blood Institute emphasizes that women with existing heart disease should not take HRT because of the increased risk of heart attack within the first few years of use, as well as an increased risk of blood clots and stroke.

While HRT seemed to be a panacea for all health problems experienced by midlife women, there are many less harmful ways of preventing heart disease than exposing yourself to the known and as-yet-unknown risks of HRT. There are also more natural ways of lowering blood pressure and reducing the risk of heart attack than using diuretics, beta-blockers, and cholesterol-lowering drugs. No matter how old we are, we need to take control of our own body and give it the optimum nutrition needed to naturally protect against hypertension and heart disease.

THE HOT TIMES APPROACH TO HEART DISEASE

You *can* significantly reduce your chances of developing heart disease by learning about the risk factors involved and making the transition to a heart-healthy lifestyle. In addition to regular exercise (see Chapter 6), a diet that is low in sodium and commercially processed oils and high in vitamins, fiber, and essential fatty acids is particularly effective in preventing heart-related illnesses. The following are some guidelines that will aid you in your quest for a strong heart and overall good health.

Dietary Recommendations: Eating for a Healthy Heart

Foods rich in the antioxidant nutrients—vitamins A, C, and E, beta-carotene, and selenium—are a must for healthy hearts. Fresh fruits, leafy green vegetables, a variety of whole grains, freshly squeezed vegetable juices, sea vegetables, garlic, and onions are good sources of these important nutrients.

Cranberries are a particularly rich source of phytonutrients that act as antioxidants, blocking the absorption of fat and lowering LDL cholesterol and triglycerides while raising HDL cholesterol. Maintain sufficient levels of vitamin D to lessen your risk of inflammation by including sardines, tuna, sweet potatoes and yams, alfalfa, and egg yolks in your diet; get plenty of sunshine; and consider taking up to 2000 IU as a supplement daily.

Follow my suggestions given earlier in this chapter to ensure you get the magnesium you need to control calcium absorption and prevent plaque formation. To control your homocysteine levels, be sure to get enough vitamins B_6 and B_{12} and folic acid. The Daily Reference Intake value for vitamin B_6 is 1.5 mg for women 50 and older. Among the best food sources are bananas, carrots, onions, asparagus, peas, sunflower seeds, walnuts, and wheat germ. The Daily Reference Intake value for vitamin B_{12} is 2.4 mcg for women 50 and older. Food sources include liver (beef and chicken), oysters, sardines, cheese, eggs, trout, salmon, and tuna. If you are vegetarian, you will have difficulty getting adequate vitamin B_{12} from your diet and may need to supplement. The Daily Reference Intake value for folic acid is 400 mcg for women 50 and older. The best food sources are green leafy vegetables, fortified yeast flakes, blue-green algae, salmon, cheese, brown rice, beef, beans, and barley. Because many people over age 50 have inadequate levels of hydrochloric acid—needed to utilize vitamin B_{12}, magnesium, and other nutrients—consider taking a hydrochloric acid supplement, especially if you have symptoms of gastric distress after eating. Look for one that includes pepsin.

Garlic with cayenne pepper is one of the best combinations for lowering blood pressure naturally. Fiber, particularly the soluble fiber found in flaxseed, fruits, vegetables, barley, and oats, helps to lower cholesterol levels and assists in eliminating toxins and carcinogens from the digestive tract.

Foods to avoid include all commercially processed oils, whole-milk dairy products, sugar, white flour, fried foods, hydrogenated fats, such as margarine and vegetable shortenings, and soybean oil. It would also be wise to limit your intake of red meat, regular salt, coffee, and alcohol.

HOLD THE SALT

Keep tabs on the sodium content of your foods to help prevent high blood pressure and stroke. Start by removing most processed foods from your diet, because they are the highest sources of sodium. This means limiting or eliminating most canned, pickled, smoked, instant, and snack foods. Dairy products are also high in sodium (unless unsalted). Become a label reader and avoid anything than contains the word *sodium* on the label, such as monosodium glutamate, sodium benzoate, sodium nitrate, and disodium phosphate. Even baking soda and baking powder are sodium-rich. Try to keep your daily sodium intake down to 2000 mg. Remember that 1 teaspoon of salt equals 2000 mg of sodium; 1 tablespoon of soy sauce contains 1029 mg of sodium.

USE HEART-SMART OILS

As you learned in this chapter, the wrong fat can be devastating for us. The right fat, however, can be healing. EFAs not only help prevent heart disease, they are vital for overall good health. Flaxseed, macadamia nut, sesame, olive, rice bran, almond, and coconut are the oils of choice in the Hot Times Diet. These oils provide us with essential and healthy fats, as well as heart-protecting nutrients—such as lecithin, beta-carotene, and vitamin E—that have been removed from processed oils.

Flaxseed oil is the best vegetable source of omega-3s, the type of fat that lowers triglyceride and bad-cholesterol levels and is most deficient in today's American diet. Flaxseed oil's incredible oxygen-absorbing ability helps to oxygenate the body. (This positive feature

should not be confused with the negative effects of oxidized cholesterol.) It's highly polyunsaturated, so it's very sensitive to light, heat,
and air. It is best used in no-heat recipes, drizzled on cooked vegetables, or as a butter substitute in hot cereals. It has a nutty, rich flavor
that may take some getting used to.

Sesame oil gets rave reviews because of its mild nutty flavor and
high versatility. It contains sesamol, a natural antioxidant that makes
it very stable and highly resistant to oxidation. It also has a fairly high
monounsaturated fat content, making it a good heart protector. This
oil is good for sautéing and baking and as a salad dressing. Give it a
try in my pungent Dilled Tofu Mustard sauce (page 253).

You're probably familiar with the virtues of olive oil, a full-bodied
oil used almost to the exclusion of other oils in the Mediterranean re-
gion, where heart disease and cancer rates are much lower than ours.
Olive oil is a monounsaturated oil, which means it is very stable
against the free-radical effects of heat, air, and light. Extra-virgin
olive oil is a wonderful oil for both cooking and using on salads. It is
a highly beneficial oil for women, because it has been shown to reduce LDL levels while keeping HDL levels high.

Three of the most stable oils, and therefore good for cooking, are
macadamia nut, rice bran, and coconut. Their stability means no
harmful trans-fatty acids or free radicals are formed when the oils are
heated. Macadamia nut oil has high levels of antioxidants and a 1:1
ratio of omega-3 to omega-6 fatty acids. Rice bran oil has a high
smoking point, and coconut oil has the additional benefits of being
antiviral and antibacterial, as well as a powerful immune system
booster.

The Woman's Oil, which I developed for Health From the Sun
and which is sold in most health food stores, contains essential fatty
acids such as omega-3–rich high-lignan flaxseed oil and omega-6–
rich black currant seed oil, and rosemary extract, which you can use
in no-heat recipes or take in capsule form as a supplement. Whenever you buy oils, look for cold expeller-pressed oils, with no chemi-

cal solvents or hydrogenation used in processing. The label should show certification as organic by an independent agency such as the Organic Crop Improvement Association. You will find many delicious ways to use these heart-smart oils in Chapter 8.

Supplements and Herbal Remedies

Hawthorn and coleus root can be effective in treating high blood pressure; hawthorn has also been found effective in relieving heart pain (angina) and rapid heartbeat (tachycardia). Always consult a knowledgeable practitioner when using herbs to treat heart disease.

Thankfully, we have made wonderful advances in recognizing the unique symptoms of heart disease in women. Controlling cholesterol levels is not enough anymore; we need to be mindful of brand-new risk factors like C-reactive protein, ferritin, and homocysteine. We can protect and heal our hearts with the right oils, minerals (like magnesium), herbs, and lifestyle habits. Heart disease—like breast cancer, diabetes, and hypothyroidism (the topics to be covered in the next chapter)—can be turned around. It's all in your hands—take heart.

FIVE

Other Midlife Concerns: Breast Cancer, Diabetes, and Hypothyroidism

As YOU MOVE INTO MIDLIFE, YOUR GREATEST FEARS MAY relate to the most common symptoms of menopause: hot flashes, sexual changes, and depression or anxiety. Although not life-threatening, these symptoms are life-altering for many of us. Thankfully, a revolution in the approach to treatment, with an emphasis on natural lifestyle modification, has proved that these discomforts—and even some of the more severe health hazards, such as osteoporosis and heart disease—are not inevitable. What you may not fully realize, however, is that you can significantly decrease your chances of developing other illnesses associated with menopause, such as breast cancer, diabetes, and hypothyroidism. These dangers can be minimized if you maintain a healthy diet and exercise program, and avoid toxic substances like tobacco and excessive amounts of alcohol.

This chapter is designed to help you understand the risks and recognize the signs of these serious health threats. Remember: Prevention is the key to beating the odds, and so I highly suggest that all Hot Times women use the recommendations in this chapter regardless of whether breast cancer, diabetes, or hypothryoidism is a current concern. I want you to be protected and therefore proactive.

BREAST CANCER

As a practicing nutritionist dealing with women's issues, I have become keenly aware over the years that many women are more terrified of breast cancer than of any other disease. Sure, more women are surviving breast cancer than in previous decades, probably because of earlier detection and improved therapies, but the occurrence rate for the disease continues to rise—up a staggering 55 percent since 1960. Despite treatment improvements, such as lumpectomies, which remove the tumor but preserve the breast, and chemotherapy combinations that may have fewer major side effects than earlier drugs, the treatment choices for this dread disease are physically and emotionally devastating. If we are to halt the rise in cases and avoid the debilitating treatments, prevention is the key.

We don't know what causes breast cancer, and the majority of breast cancer cases occur in women with no known risk factors. Nevertheless, research continues to find associations between breast cancer and a variety of factors. As with heart disease, some risk factors for breast cancer are beyond our control. For example, an estimated 10 percent of cases are linked to inherited gene mutations, but these cancers occur primarily before menopause. Breast cancer occurring after menopause is more commonly the result of lifestyle influences such as diet and environment, which we have the ability to change. The incidence rises sharply in women after age 40, with 77 percent of invasive breast cancer occurring in women 50 and older. Breast cancer strikes white women more often than women of color. In addition, the following five characteristics have been identified by researchers as common in women who develop breast cancer:

- a mother or sister who has had breast cancer
- having had cancer in one breast
- never having borne a child and being past the age to do so

- being over thirty at the time of your first pregnancy
- beginning menstruation early (before the age of 12) or entering menopause late (after the age of 55)

This does not necessarily mean that if you fit one or more of these characteristics you will get breast cancer, but the risk is there.

Researchers have found that estrogen, in particular estradiol and estrone, stimulates breast cancer cell growth, which probably accounts for the length of menstruation being a risk factor. This probably also explains the significant risk of developing breast cancer for women who take hormone replacement therapy (HRT). As I noted previously, the Women's Health Initiative study of two types of HRT was halted before completion because of an unacceptable level of breast cancer in women taking HRT, particularly within the first three years. Moreover, the cancer tended to be found at a more advanced stage. Another study from the United Kingdom found women taking HRT who developed breast cancer were more likely to die of the disease than were women who weren't on the hormone therapy. Finally, in 2004, a Swedish study of menopausal women who were taking HRT after surviving breast cancer was also halted, because, as the researchers concluded, even short-term use of hormone therapy poses an unacceptably high risk of breast cancer.

On the other hand, two hormones appear to have a protective effect when it comes to breast cancer. Both progesterone (the natural hormone, not the synthetic progestin) and the third estrogen, estriol, have been shown to slow cell growth.

Clearly, your level of estrogen from HRT is a risk factor over which you have control. Weight is another. Menopausal women who are overweight have an increased risk of breast cancer. Fat tissue can convert other hormones into estrogen, increasing your estrogen levels. In addition, obese women are more likely to develop insulin resistance and diabetes, both of which are associated with higher risks of breast cancer. As with heart disease, if you accumulate fat at your waist (apple-shaped), you are at greater risk than if you accumulate fat at your hips and thighs (pear-shaped).

Yet another risk factor you can control is the type and amount of fat you consume. If you are like most Americans, your diet contains excess saturated fats and trans-fatty acids and too few of the powerful omega-3 fatty acids. Trans fats produce damaging free radicals in your body, while omega-3 fatty acids protect your body from the cancer-promoting actions of arachidonic acid.

Lack of exercise also appears to increase your risk. Exercising regularly for about four hours a week gives you one-third to one-half the chance of developing breast cancer than if you are sedentary. As I discuss in greater detail in the next chapter, exercise stimulates your lymphatic system. This intricate system of channels and nodes lying just underneath your skin is responsible for ridding your body of toxins that mimic estrogens, fat globules, toxic waste products from metabolism, dead cells, and heavy metals. Exercise also keeps insulin levels low and helps control weight, further reducing your breast cancer risk.

A link between smoking and breast cancer has not yet been conclusively shown, although some studies indicate an increased risk for women who began smoking in early adolescence. On the other hand, women who drink as few as two alcoholic drinks a day have one and one-half times the breast cancer risk of women who drink no alcohol.

Making the lifestyle changes you'll find in Hot Times can go far toward lowering your risk of developing breast cancer, but you still need to take advantage of all the tools available for early diagnosis. There are many books available that deal with the diagnosis and treatment of breast cancer. I encourage you to learn and practice breast self-examination. The American Cancer Society suggests women practice breast examination about a week after the end of their menstrual period. For those past menopause, examine the first day of each month. Your doctor's office or your local American Cancer Society chapter can provide you with information on how to do your own breast examination.

A second early-detection method is mammograms. These breast X-rays can spotlight small growths that cannot be found through self-examination. The American Cancer Society recommends a baseline mammogram at age 35. A mammogram is recommended every two years after age 40; after age 50, every year. Remember to include supplemental antioxidants—particularly extra vitamin C, vitamin A, and selenium the day before, the day of, and the day after a mammogram. This will protect you against free radicals from X-ray exposure.

Mammography is not without its problems, of course. Although radiation levels have been reduced in modern devices, you nevertheless are being exposed to potentially harmful radiation. If you have large or dense breasts, your mammogram results may be unreliable. As with any diagnostic test, mammography produces some false results—about 30 percent of positive results and 10 to 20 percent of negative readings are incorrect, causing delays in treatment, inappropriate treatment, and unnecessary anxiety. Mammograms also can only detect actual tumors, not the precancerous cells that are present before a tumor actually forms.

For all these reasons, many research studies are under way to find other, more effective screening tools. One of the more promising tests is thermography, also known as digital infrared thermal imaging. Cancerous cells often develop additional blood vessels to increase the blood flow to provide the nutrients they need to grow; this additional flow generates heat that can be detected by thermography's highly sensitive infrared cameras and then used to produce images. Thus, thermography can detect areas of precancerous cells without radiation or invasive procedures. However, at present, it doesn't work well with slow-growing tumors or ones that don't develop their own blood vessels, and it isn't precise enough to pinpoint the location of tumors. By combining both mammography and thermography, a woman has about a 95 percent chance of detecting significant changes. Thermography isn't available everywhere, but you may be able to locate a clinic if you ask your doctor or check at www.breastthermography.com.

The Hot Times Approach to Breast Cancer

High-fat diets have been implicated in breast cancer. After carefully reviewing the studies, however, I believe it's more a question of the kind of fat consumed than the amount. Women in Mediterranean countries show a low level of breast cancer yet consume a high-fat diet (40 percent of total calories); the key seems to be that the fat they consume is monounsaturated olive oil. Animal studies have confirmed that when test animals are fed olive oil–rich diets, they show fewer breast tumors than animals on a high–polyunsaturated fat diet. Japanese women, eating their native diets, consume fat in the form of cold-water fish (salmon, mackeral, and sardines), a rich source of omega-3 fatty acids. Their breast cancer rates are four times less than American women. Once these Japanese start eating a Western diet, which includes different kinds of fat, they begin to show cancer rates nearer the higher American levels. Greenland Inuit, whose diets are uncommonly high in fat (also in the form of fish oils), rarely develop breast cancer.

KNOW YOUR FATS

Worried about cholesterol and fat, many women have dramatically reduced their consumption of artery-clogging saturated fats from whole milk, red meat, and eggs. Although they seem to be reducing fat intake, the truth is they have merely shifted their source of fat from saturated to commercially processed polyunsaturated fat or hydrogenated fat found in corn, safflower, soybean oil, or margarine, which are touted by advertisers to lower cholesterol.

But these seemingly healthful polyunsaturated substitutes may actually be worse for the female breast. Breast tumors appeared more frequently in laboratory animals fed diets high in safflower and corn oil than in those fed olive oil. In addition, researchers have noted dramatically higher levels of toxic chemicals such as dichlorodiphenyltrichloroethane (DDT) and polychlorinated biphenyls (PCBs) in women with breast cancer. So again, it may not be simply the fat in the diet but what is in the fat. Toxic environmental wastes are stored in fatty tissue, and the breast is a primary fatty tissue in women. This means organically grown food is your best bet.

Among the best oils are flaxseed, perilla, olive, macadamia nut, rice bran, and sesame. Flaxseed oil is one of the richest sources of omega-3 fatty acid. To match the omega-3 power of two tablespoons of flaxseed oil, you would need to eat nearly two pounds of albacore tuna. Flaxseed oil is particularly female-friendly because it contains high levels of alpha-linolenic acid, making it superior to fish oils, which contain none. A recent French study found that women with high levels of alpha-linolenic acid in their adipose breast tissue had a 60 percent lower risk of breast cancer than women with low levels of the fatty acid.

Flaxseed is also a rich source of the phytonutrient lignans, containing as much as 800 times more lignans than wheat bran, oats, or soybeans. Lignans help remove excess estrogen from the body by binding with estrogen receptors. According to research from the University of Toronto, this antiestrogen effect of flaxseed was stronger than that of soy—yet another reason to choose flaxseed over soy. Lignans are found in the shell of the flaxseed, so when you buy flaxseed oil, look for one that is labeled high-lignan flaxseed oil, in which tiny particles of lignan-containing seed husk are held in suspension in the oil. The oil has a nutty flavor and quickly becomes rancid in heat, light, or oxygen, so I suggest using it as a salad dressing or drizzling it on steamed vegetables or other side dishes. Refrigerate the bottle after opening. One or two tablespoons a day is enough to give you the healthful benefits.

For low-temperature cooking, centuries of Mediterranean cooks know olive oil is a cancer-smart choice. This monounsaturated oil has numerous healthful benefits, among them apparently as a breast cancer preventive. Harvard researchers have found that women who consumed olive oil more than twice a day had a 25 percent lower risk of developing breast cancer.

Some of the most stable oils, and therefore good for cooking, are macadamia nut, rice bran, and coconut. Their stability means no harmful trans-fatty acids or free radicals are formed when the oils are heated. Macadamia nut oil has high levels of antioxidants and an ideal 1:1 ratio of omega-3 to omega-6 fatty acids. It gives a delightful flavor to my Almond Sunrise Pancakes (page 199). Rice bran oil has a rather delicate flavor and a very high smoking point, so it can be used for frying. Coconut oil has the additional benefits of being antiviral and antibacterial, as well as a powerful immune system booster. Because of its saturated fat content, however, coconut oil should be used in moderation, such as in my special occasion Carrot Cake for a Crowd (page 284).

Whenever you buy oils, look for cold expeller-pressed oils with no chemical solvents or hydrogenation used in processing. The label should show certification as organic by an independent agency such as the Organic Crop Improvement Association. You will find many delicious ways to use these cancer-fighting oils in Chapter 8.

THE IMPORTANCE OF FIBER

Researchers have also observed an association between accumulated waste materials in the intestinal tract and toxic accumulations in women's breasts. The buildup of waste in the intestinal tract is due in large part to a diet lacking in fiber. Fiber is the nonnutritive element in plant foods that is indigestible by the human body. It speeds the time it takes food to pass through the intestinal tract, so noxious wastes are removed from the system quickly. Food that remains in the intestinal tract too long can ferment and putrefy, producing toxic chemicals that are released into the bloodstream. In women, these wastes can eventually get dumped in breast tissue. The buildup of waste materials in the intestine can result from simple constipation, and an association between constipation and breast cancer has also been seen. Therefore, increasing fiber in your diet to keep your system "swept out" helps to prevent the accumulation of toxic wastes in the intestine as well as in the breast tissue.

In the 1960s, British doctors who studied African populations discovered a strong relationship between high fiber intake and a low rate of degenerative diseases. Because of the enormous amount of refined and processed foods we consume, the average American diet contains only between 8 and 11 grams of fiber; the recommended daily requirement is between 20 and 30 grams. Lack of dietary fiber has been linked to a whole host of diseases common in Western society, such as heart disease, diabetes, high blood pressure, hemorrhoids, varicose veins, food allergies, and various cancers, including breast cancer.

Insoluble fibers from flaxseed, for example, absorb water in your digestive tract, speeding the removal of waste products. Increase fiber-rich whole grains, fruits, and vegetables in your diet; eat five servings a day of a variety of fruits and vegetables. Eat fruits and vegetables in their whole form rather than juice, and leave the peels on as much as possible, as the skins contain fiber and other nutrients.

CANCER-FIGHTING FRUITS AND VEGETABLES

The cruciferous vegetables—including broccoli, bok choy, cauliflower, Brussels sprouts, and cabbage—are rich sources of a nitrogen-like compound called indole. The indole compound is believed to help deactivate excess estrogen in the body, which fuels cancer. Beta-carotene–rich foods also appear to be powerful cancer fighters. Carrots, squash, sweet potatoes, yams, cantaloupes, peaches, and dark green leafy vegetables—such as kale, collard, spinach, and mustard greens—all contain healthy amounts of beta-carotene.

Boost your intake of antioxidants by eating cranberries, which contain phytonutrients such as anthocyanins and luteins. I believe that these nutrients have the ability to digest fatty globules in the lymph to help keep it functioning properly. Another antioxidant that has been strongly associated with lower breast cancer risk is lycopene, found in cooked tomatoes. Antioxidants neutralize the effects of damaging free radicals. While it is preferable to get your antioxidants from fruits, vegetables, and other foods, you may need to supplement daily to ensure you are getting enough of these cancer-fighting nutrients: vitamin C (75 mg), vitamin E (400 IU), and selenium (55 mcg).

VITAMIN D

Most people are aware of vitamin D's role in bone health but may be less aware of recent research that has linked vitamin D deficiencies to breast, prostate, colon, and skin cancers, and to increased inflammation in otherwise healthy people, contributing to heart disease, arthritis, and diabetes. Up to 85 percent of American adults may be vitamin D–deficient, particularly older people, and need to get at least 1000 to 2000 IU daily, primarily from supplements. In addition to adequate exposure to sunlight, sources of vitamin D include sardines, tuna, sweet potatoes and yams, alfalfa, and egg yolks.

THE MANY BENEFITS OF GARLIC

Garlic is an age-old, time-honored remedy, used for centuries for myriad health problems. Only recently has science begun to pay the respect due this "stinking rose." A whole host of research studies show garlic to be beneficial in lowering cholesterol, controlling infection, boosting immunity, protecting your body from environmental pollution, and lowering blood sugar, as well as preventing cancer. Specific to breast cancer, aged garlic extracts have been shown to inhibit the growth of breast cancer cells in the test tube. Garlic, incorporated in cooking or taken as a prepared extract, just may give us an easy ounce of prevention for breast cancer.

WHAT TO AVOID

Synthetic hormones such as diethylstilbesterol (DES), used to stimulate growth in food stocks, are forms of estrogen. Residues remain in meat, and eating large quantities assures you get a hefty dose of secondhand drugs. Residues, as I have mentioned, have a tendency to be stored in fatty tissues, especially the breasts. You should avoid all meat and poultry products that have been deliberately fed or implanted with synthetic hormones to speed growth. Look for hormone- and antibiotic-free meat and poultry from organic producers. Many of my clients have reported more energy when they eat organically grown lean red meat once or twice a week. Organically raised poultry should be consumed in place of commercially raised poultry as much as possible.

Both animal and human research studies have found associations between high-sugar diets and increased rates of breast cancer, particularly in women over 45. Cancer cells need as much as ten times more glucose to thrive than do normal cells, so an important step in prevention is passing over highly sweetened processed foods, soft drinks, fruit juices, and, of course, the sugar bowl.

Painful lumps in the breasts, known as fibrocystic breast disease or benign breast disease, affect 60 percent of all women during their lives. Although not considered a risk factor for breast cancer, the condition creates fear in women nevertheless. Diets high in caffeine and the related chemical methylxanthine from coffee, sodas, chocolate, cocoa, and tea have been strongly connected to fibrocystic breast disease. I have found that when my clients totally removed caffeine and caffeine-related foods, even decaffeinated coffee, from their diet, their painful breast lumps disappeared. Breast lumps have been found to be dramatically reduced by the intake of 600 IU of vitamin E daily. The topical use of natural progesterone cream also reduces breast cysts.

DIABETES AND OTHER BLOOD
SUGAR DISORDERS

In the late 1980s, the U.S. surgeon general and the USDA issued new dietary guidelines in the form of a food pyramid to try to control the rising incidence of heart disease, obesity, and diabetes. Twenty-five years later, the food pyramid has been a dismal failure. Americans interpreted the pyramid's reliance on carbohydrates as a rationale for continuing to consume huge quantities of processed, simple carbohydrates, not the complex carbs the scientists intended. These processed foods may have been fat-free, but they were full of sugar, white flour, and sodium.

Between 1997 and 2002, the percent of Americans diagnosed with diabetes increased 27 percent. About 12 million American adults have been diagnosed and another 5 million have the disease but are unaware of it. Diabetes is the fifth leading cause of death for women and carries with it a wide range of serious complications, including heart disease, kidney failure, and blindness. African-Americans, Latinos, Native Americans, and Asian-Americans/Pacific Islanders are particularly at risk to develop the disease.

Diabetes is actually one of several conditions that results from malfunctions in the body's system to regulate glucose. Glucose is the form of sugar carried in your bloodstream and is used by every cell for energy. After you eat, blood glucose levels rise, causing, in healthy individuals, a reaction of the pancreas to secrete insulin, the hormone that carries the glucose to the cells. Glucose that is not immediately needed is converted to glycogen and stored in the liver and muscles. When additional energy is needed, the liver converts the glycogen back to glucose.

In response to large quantities of glucose—from breads, flour- or sugar-based snack foods, and sweets—the pancreas produces large quantities of insulin. For reasons not fully understood, the insulin receptors on each cell develop resistance to these floods of insulin.

Glucose cannot enter the cells, so it remains in the bloodstream, where it stimulates even more insulin. Chronically high insulin promotes abdominal fat storage, raises blood pressure, and worsens blood fat profiles. When the prediabetic condition of insulin resistance is accompanied by obesity, high blood pressure, high triglycerides, or high cholesterol, the condition is known as Syndrome X, a significant risk factor for heart disease. If the pancreas is forced to continue to produce insulin, eventually its beta cells become exhausted, insulin production is insufficient, and type 2 diabetes results.

Type 2 diabetes (formerly known as adult-onset or non–insulin-dependent diabetes) is the most common of several forms of diabetes. Type 1 diabetes, once known as juvenile-onset or insulin-dependent diabetes, results when little or no insulin is produced by the pancreas. It is usually diagnosed in childhood and is believed to be an autoimmune disease often triggered by a virus or bacteria. Insulin injections and careful dietary monitoring are needed for the rest of the diabetic's life. Gestational diabetes develops in women during pregnancy and usually disappears after the birth.

One of the most promising areas of diabetes research concerns the role of inflammation in type 2 diabetes. In women, researchers have found an association between higher levels of the inflammation marker C-reactive protein (CRP) and the onset of Syndrome X and type 2 diabetes. When blood sugar levels are high, CRP is especially active in stimulating an enzyme that interferes with the breakdown of blood clots. This process appears to cause damage to your arteries that leads to plaque buildup and more clots. Animal studies have found that in the presence of chronic inflammation, insulin use becomes less efficient and diabetes results. There may even be a role for weight gain in this inflammatory process. It seems that, like immune cells, fat cells release cytokines, which stimulate an immune response and cause inflammation. These fat cells are particularly active as you gain weight. (For more on inflammation and disease, see Chapter 4.)

Among the better-known risk factors for developing type 2 diabetes are

- obesity, especially when fat is carried at the abdomen (apple shape)
- diet high in sugar and simple carbohydrates
- stress, which stimulates cortisol with its tendency to encourage abdominal fat
- hypothyroidism, resulting in less thyroxine being available to increase the response to insulin (see later in this chapter)
- lack of exercise
- gender and age, with women over 45 twice as likely to develop diabetes as men

High blood sugar is also a side effect of taking a number of medications, including calcium channel blockers, antihypertensives, corticosteroids, thyroid medications, and certain anticonvulsant drugs. If you fall into one of these risk categories for diabetes, you should take steps outlined in the Hot Times Approach to Diabetes.

The major symptoms of type 2 diabetes include constant thirst, frequent nighttime urination, excessive fatigue, poor circulation, and unexplained weight loss. If you suspect you may have diabetes, contact your doctor immediately. Diabetes can be medically diagnosed by a fasting blood test that measures blood sugar levels. It is generally recommended to take the test twice, at least several days apart. A glucose reading greater than 126 mg per 100 ml of blood is considered diagnostic for diabetes. Anyone with a blood sugar level between 110 and 125 mg per 100 ml is considered prediabetic.

The Hot Times Approach to Diabetes

Because diabetes is caused by an inability to metabolize glucose, diet is the crucial preventive and treatment measure and the focus of the

Hot Times approach. By simply controlling the amount of sugar you consume, you can control the available glucose in your bloodstream. And by consuming fiber, protein, cinnamon, and acidic foods, you can actually control the pace at which glucose is released. You can also keep insulin levels low by eating foods rich in omega-3 fatty acids. Certain vitamins and minerals can also help balance both insulin and glucose in your bloodstream.

Regulating your sugar consumption is crucial in the prevention and control of diabetes. Eliminate all products high in sugar and white flour, such as cookies, cakes, pies, ice cream, candy, and pastries. Even concentrated carbohydrates from natural sources, such as honey and fruit juices, are a constant challenge to the pancreas.

FIBER

Fiber is a key element in your diet to combat diabetes. Limit your intake of processed and refined carbohydrates and instead emphasize more complex carbohydrates from flaxseed, vegetables, fruits, beans, and whole grains in your diet. These provide a greater amount of fiber, which helps your body slow the release of sugar into your bloodstream. I suggest three or more servings per day of these fiber-rich foods. At the same time, be sure to increase your water intake to help move the fiber through the intestines. If you don't drink enough liquid, fiber can cause constipation.

OMEGA-3 FATTY ACIDS

In addition to all the benefits described in the chapters on other midlife conditions, consuming omega-3 fatty acids appears to contribute to enhanced insulin sensitivity. By increasing HDL (good) cholesterol, decreasing triglycerides, and lowering blood pressure, omega-3 fatty acids also help reverse Syndrome X, contributing to improved heart health at the same time. Flaxseed oil is one of the best sources of omega-3. Adding the oil to your diet causes your stomach to retain food for a longer period of time, resulting in a slow, sustained rise in blood sugar rather than a sharp spike. On the other hand, excessive nonessential fats, especially those found in full-fat dairy products, such as butter, cheese, and ice cream, block insulin activity in the blood.

PROTEIN

An easy way to reduce your craving for sweets when following a Hot Times Diet is to keep your protein levels steady. Protein stimulates the pancreas to produce glucagon. For this reason, I suggest you include at least two 3½-ounce servings of fish, poultry, and other foods high in protein (low-fat cheese, beans, tempeh) each day, including up to four eggs per week. Eat lean red meat (hormone-free) once or twice a week. Refer to Chapter 7 for the complete food plan and menus.

HERBS

Herbalists have used cedar berries and blueberry leaf (as a tea) for centuries to help control diabetes. Cinnamon, about one-quarter teaspoon per day, can also help diabetics by keeping glucose levels steady. Research at the USDA's Human Nutrition Research Center has shown that cinnamon helps insulin to metabolize blood sugar with twenty times greater efficiency. Cloves, bay leaf, coriander, cayenne, dry mustard, and ginger are all healthy spices that can decrease your risk of excess insulin by either speeding your metabolism or lowering glucose levels.

ACIDIC FOODS

Acidic foods such as lemon juice and apple cider vinegar have been shown to lower blood sugar by up to 30 percent by slowing digestion of carbohydrates. Enjoy the benefits of some acidic ingredients with my Herb-Crusted Salmon Fillet (page 263) or in my salad dressing recipes (page 227).

MINERALS

Two specific minerals, zinc and chromium, act as insulin cofactors and should be taken as supplements by diabetics or by those at risk for diabetes. Zinc forms part of the insulin component secreted by the pancreas and is directly involved in the body's metabolism of carbohydrates; it also has a powerful influence on wound healing and disease resistance, two factors important for diabetics, who can suffer from impaired healing and lowered immunity. Some of the best sources of zinc are lean red meats, eggs, pumpkin seeds, seafood (particularly oysters), dried beans, and legumes. A supplement containing 25 mg of zinc should be considered if you are not fond of these foods.

Chromium, an essential trace mineral, is absolutely necessary for proper insulin function, because it regulates the metabolism of sugar. This mineral is useful for both diabetics and hypoglycemics (those with low blood sugar). In animal studies, chromium deficiency was shown to cause diabetes and was reversed with the addition of chromium. In human diabetics, ingestion of chromium resulted in the normalization of glucose tolerance tests in 50 percent of the patients tested. New studies suggest chromium helps control hunger, burns calories, and, in athletes, increases endurance and assists in gaining muscle and losing fat. Yet nine out of ten Americans are deficient in this critical mineral, as food processing and chromium-depleted soils leave little of this mineral available to us through food. The best food sources seem to be broccoli, brown rice, oysters, mushrooms, and whole grains. I suggest dietary supplements (at least 200 mcg once or twice a day with meals) to assure adequate levels, because most people don't eat enough chromium-rich foods.

A third mineral, magnesium, has been shown to improve insulin sensitivity in people with type 2 diabetes. In addition, researchers at Johns Hopkins University found low blood levels of magnesium to be a predictor of type 2 diabetes. Sources of magnesium include leafy green vegetables, kale, celery, alfalfa sprouts, beans, seeds, and nuts. Most women will also need to supplement with 500 mg a day.

VITAMINS

Women with diabetes need more vitamin C than other people because without enough insulin, the vitamin doesn't get into the cells. One study found that when women with diabetes took 2000 mg of vitamin C a day, their blood sugar levels dropped (as did their cholesterol and triglycerides). Include vitamin C–rich foods in your diet every day, such as citrus fruit, strawberries, bell peppers, tomatoes, Brussels sprouts, cauliflower, broccoli, cabbage, and spinach.

Because vitamin D deficiency has been associated with C-reactive protein and inflammation that can contribute to diabetes, women should take 1000 to 2000 IU daily, along with getting plenty of sunshine and eating vitamin D–rich foods such as sardines, tuna, sweet potatoes and yams, alfalfa, and egg yolks.

EXERCISE

Finally, the couch potatoes among you have yet another reason to start exercising. A recent study from the Diabetes Prevention Program demonstrated that thirty minutes a day of moderate physical activity, such as I describe in the next chapter, combined with a 5 to 10 percent reduction in body weight, produced a 58 percent reduction in diabetes in people with prediabetic insulin resistance.

Hypothyroidism

A member of the endocrine system of glands, the thyroid is a small butterfly-shaped gland in the neck, just below the Adam's apple. Although it weighs less than 1 ounce and secretes less than 1 teaspoon of thyroid hormone a year, it is pivotal in regulating the body's metabolism. The thyroid hormone thyroxine keeps all bodily processes operating, including heart rate, body temperature, muscle contraction, calorie use, protein synthesis, and production of the enzymes used to break down carbohydrates to glucose.

Thyroid problems are common—more common than many health professionals recognize—especially among Hot Times women. Low thyroid function, known as hypothyroidism, affects as many as 27 million Americans. Women are eight times more likely than men to suffer from hypothyroidism, most commonly developing symptoms between the ages of 35 and 60.

Unfortunately, many of the symptoms are often subtle and non-specific, making it difficult to diagnose. Common symptoms include

- fatigue
- intolerance to cold
- cold hands and feet
- loss of appetite
- weight gain
- swelling around the eyes
- muscle weakness and cramping
- aching wrists, arms, and hands
- depression
- insomnia
- irritability
- inability to concentrate
- premature graying of hair
- hair loss
- inappropriate hair growth
- dry, scaly skin
- brittle nails
- hot flashes
- menstrual irregularities
- fluid retention
- decreased libido
- constipation

- difficulty swallowing pills/lump in throat
- coarse voice

You probably noticed that many of these symptoms are also associated with menopause. Unfortunately, women may be prescribed hormone replacement therapy to relieve menopause symptoms that are
really signs of hypothyroidism. Excess estrogen produces a protein
that binds to thyroid hormone and prevents it from fully functioning.

The causes of hypothydroidism are varied. Several medical conditions and their treatments can result in hypothyroidism—for example, surgery or radiation treatment for Graves' disease and thyroid
cancer. Corticosteroids, cholesterol-lowering drugs, antidepressants,
and certain other medications can affect thyroid function either by
blocking hormone production or by binding to the hormone and limiting its effectiveness.

Because thyroid gland function is closely intertwined with that of
the adrenal glands (see Chapter 2), the thyroid and adrenals compete
for the amino acid tyrosine to produce their hormones. Under stress,
the adrenals may use the available tyrosine to make cortisol, depriving the thyroid of the supply it needs to make its hormones. Under
conditions of adrenal burnout, the thyroid will work harder to stimulate adrenal activity, until it, too, becomes exhausted, resulting in
hypothyroidism.

Dietary factors can also trigger hypothyroidism. Iodine is an ingredient in two thyroid hormones, and too much or too little can lead to
low thyroid function. Unfortunately, depletion of iodine in soils and
low consumption of iodized salt and high-iodine foods such as sea
vegetables have resulted in deficiencies. (To test your iodine levels,
see page 147.) Overdoing soy, particularly for people with a family
history of thyroid disease, who have had previous thyroid problems,
or who are iodine-deficient, may trigger poor thyroid function. Certain
raw vegetables, such as Brussels sprouts, rutabaga, turnips, radishes,

cauliflower, millet, cabbage, and kale, may also lower thyroid function. Cooking these vegetables, or consuming them moderately when raw, can help protect you from their effects on your thyroid. Hypothyroidism may actually be an autoimmune disease in some people. For reasons not yet fully understood, the immune system begins attacking thyroid gland cells and their enzymes as foreign bodies. Hashimoto's thyroiditis is one of the most common forms of autoimmune hypothyroidism. If your thyroid becomes inflamed from a viral infection, the gland may release its entire store of hormones into the blood at one time. This causes a brief period of overactivity (hyperthyroidism), but quickly results in low thyroid function.

An often overlooked factor in low thyroid function is systemic candidiasis. *Candida albicans* is a yeastlike fungus, naturally occurring in our bodies. *Candida* only becomes a problem when it grows out of control and out of balance with the bacteria in our bodies. Overgrowth of *Candida* is prevalent among women who have a history of antibiotic use, have been on estrogen therapy (including birth control pills), have had children, and/or have consumed high-sugar diets. As many as one in three women may have an overgrowth of *Candida*. The fungus protein binds to the thyroid hormone, making it unavailable.

As you might expect, malfunctions of a gland so central to the workings of every cell in our body can bring on other serious diseases. Insufficient thyroxine means fat metabolism is slowed, resulting in elevated levels of total cholesterol and triglycerides. Even borderline hypothyroidism, referred to as functional hypothyroidism, is associated with high blood pressure in menopausal women. A recent Swiss study found that people with low thyroid function had increased levels of C-reactive protein, and people with more severe hypothyroidism developed high levels of homocysteine as well. As you'll remember from my discussion on heart disease, all of these factors—raised cholesterol, triglycerides, blood pressure, C-reactive protein, and homocysteine—are known to increase your risk of developing heart disease.

When thyroid function slows, the risk of osteoporosis increases for at least two reasons. First, low thyroid function means inadequate calcitonin, a hormone necessary for balancing the levels of calcium in the blood, is produced. It's calcitonin that blocks bone breakdown and encourages calcium assimilation from the blood. Second, hypothyroidism blocks production of hydrochloric acid in the stomach. As I discussed in Chapter 3, hydrochloric acid creates the proper pH within the stomach to ensure breakdown of calcium and its cofactors so they can be used for bone-building.

Hypothyroidism also appears to reduce the number of insulin receptors in the liver, thus contributing to insulin resistance. Your thyroid gland works along with your pancreas and liver to keep blood sugar levels stable. When blood sugar levels are low, thyroxine stimulates the conversion of protein and fats to glycogen; high blood sugar levels cause thyroxine to help convert glucose to glycogen for storage. The lack of thyroxine leads to a sluggish immune system, leaving your body vulnerable to recurring infections and a host of autoimmune disorders.

One of the more accurate tests for thyroid function is the basal temperature test, developed by Broda O. Barnes, M.D., Ph.D., a pioneer in thyroid research and the author of *Hypothyroidism: The Unsuspected Illness*. This simple test involves taking the axillary (underarm) temperature before rising on consecutive mornings. Because of temperature fluctuations during the menstrual cycle, women should take this test on the second and third days of their period. At night, before retiring, shake down a thermometer and lay it beside the bed on a night table or chair. On awakening in the morning, before getting out of bed, place the thermometer under your bare arm for ten minutes. Record the temperature for two consecutive days. The temperature range for normal thyroid function is 97.8°F to 98.2°F. A reading below this range is strongly suggestive of low thyroid function. Readings above this range may indicate infection or an overactive thyroid gland.

The standard blood tests for thyroid function used by most doctors to measure the two types of thyroxine in your bloodstream, T3 and T4, are not sensitive enough in many cases. But if you and your doctor decide to have blood tests done, insist that you have the full range of five tests performed. Most doctors rely on the TSH blood test; this measures the level of thyroid-stimulating hormone being secreted by your pituitary. (If your thyroid is functioning properly, your pituitary gland secretes very little TSH, giving you a low score on the test.) Unfortunately, relying solely on this test may identify only 2 to 5 percent of people with hypothyroidism.

Your body requires adequate levels of iodine in order to function properly. To test your iodine levels, use a cotton swab dipped in 2 percent tincture of iodine (available at most drugstores and supermarkets). Paint a silver dollar–sized spot on your abdomen or thigh. Allow it to dry before replacing your clothing. Check it frequently. If the spot remains visible for twenty-four hours, you have adequate supplies of iodine for your thyroid to function. You are iodine-deficient if the stain disappears in less than twenty-four hours. One way to replenish the supply is to continue painting a spot as soon as you notice the previous spot has disappeared. Once the stain remains for twenty-four hours (which may take several weeks), your iodine level has stabilized.

The Hot Times Approach to Hypothyroidism

Fortunately, nutrition can go a long way in helping the thyroid. Of all the raw materials used by the thyroid, iodine is probably the one you are familiar with, because it is the most well known, but many other nutrients, including the B vitamins, zinc, manganese, and the amino acids phenylalanine and tyrosine, are essential for proper functioning of this important gland.

DIET

Thyroid-blocking foods—such as soy, particularly fermented soy products, and uncooked cabbage, cauliflower, mustard greens, turnips, Brussels sprouts, kale, and rutabaga—should be avoided, not only by those on synthetic thyroid hormones but also by any woman who suspects she may have thyroid problems. If you have *Candida*, limit all yeast-containing and fermented foods, alcohol, and sugar. Nourishing the thyroid, whether you are taking medication or not, will help to correct underlying vitamin and mineral imbalances and strengthen this primary gland. As you supplement nutritionally, your need for medication may decrease. Remember to check with your physician to make sure you are not overmedicating a condition that has been nutritionally corrected.

Low thyroid function interferes with the proper absorption of the essential fatty acids, so I recommend that Hot Times women include black currant seed oil for omega-6 EFA and flaxseed oil for omega-3 EFA every day. This is one of the main reasons I developed the Woman's Oil, which combines both oils in a balanced ratio, along with vitamin E and plant nutrients, to make getting these EFAs easy and effective. For cooking, use olive oil, macadamia nut, or rice bran oil. Coconut oil is believed to increase metabolism and raise basal body temperature, which can be helpful for those with low thyroid function.

VITAMINS AND MINERALS

Correcting underlying vitamin and mineral imbalances can do much to correct thyroid function without use of the synthetic hormones traditionally prescribed. Nourish your thyroid by eating vitamin B–rich foods such as wheat germ, whole grains, nuts, seeds, dark green leafy vegetables, and legumes. Sea vegetables (such as kelp, dulse, and Irish moss), eggs, cold-water fish (salmon, mackerel, and sardines), and natural iodized salt are good sources of iodine. Vitamin E is essential for increasing iodine absorption and can be taken along with it in the form of wheat germ oil (the richest natural source) or vitamin E supplements. Foods, such as meat, poultry, fish, legumes, nuts, eggs, whole-wheat bread, and cheese, that have particularly high concentrations of the amino acid phenylalanine will enhance hormone function.

Because so many women find it hard to get all the nutrients they need for healthy thyroid function from their diet (even with my great Hot Times recipes), as I mentioned before, I've developed the Female Multiple supplement (Uni Key), with most of the vitamins and minerals needed for good thyroid function, even iodine. If you prefer to take individual supplements, other nutritional experts and the USDA suggest the following daily levels: vitamin A, 700 IU; vitamin B_2 (riboflavin), 1.1 mg; vitamin B_6, 1.5 mg; vitamin E, 400 IU; zinc, 8 mg; iron, 8 mg; selenium, 55 mcg; and iodine, 150 mcg. Add a 250 mg tyrosine and 1-2 hydrochloric acid supplements, especially if you are prone to digestive disorders.

The minerals calcium, magnesium, sodium, and potassium also help to regulate thyroid function. The thyroid hormones manufactured in your body need both iodine and phenylalanine (which breaks down into tyrosine). Low levels of zinc and phenylalanine have also been shown to reduce levels of thyroid hormones. For those who suspect they may need help with thyroid function, I would suggest taking at least 25 mg of zinc on a daily basis for one month, then reducing to 15 mg for three times per week thereafter.

One of the best noninvasive ways to find out which particular vitamins and minerals you may be deficient in is through a special test called a hair analysis, which measures tissue mineral levels. Your hair, considered a storage organ, gives a better picture of underlying nutrient imbalances than your blood, because hair can reveal what has been going on in your body for several months. (See the Resource section, page 289.)

There are effective nutritional strategies that can help to prevent and treat breast cancer, diabetes, and hypothyroidism. The Hot Times approach for these concerns, and other health issues at this time of life, definitely puts you in the driver's seat when managing your health. The only thing that may be missing from your Hot Times prescription is coming up in the next chapter—exercise.

SIX

The Hot Times Exercise Prescription

EXERCISE AND A BALANCED DIET ARE THE TWO MOST IM-portant lifestyle habits for the Hot Times woman. Exercise helps our bodies keep off the weight, allows us to better handle stress, and reduces the risks of osteoporosis and heart disease. Everybody can exercise in one way or another.

Exercise is beneficial to the body in numerous ways. It brings blood, nutrients, and fresh oxygen to every cell in the body. It improves digestion, absorption, metabolism, and assimilation of food, while increasing the efficiency of the body's enzyme reserves. For midlife women, it is a wonderful way of lowering blood fats, while keeping the good, HDL (high-density lipoprotein) cholesterol elevated. For diabetics and women with insulin resistance, exercise can lower blood sugar levels and make insulin more effective for your muscle and fat cells. Recent research has found that women who exercise regularly for about four hours a week have one-third to one-half the chance of developing breast cancer.

Regular exercise increases endurance, muscle tone and strength, flexibility, and disease resistance. The cardiovascular system is particularly benefited: As the lungs and heart become stronger, arteries become more resilient, blood pressure is lowered, and blood lipid levels of both cholesterol and triglycerides are controlled. Because exercise encourages increased blood flow, it is a strong weapon against many midlife health problems, including strokes, atherosclerosis, phlebitis, and heart attacks. Joint problems such as bursitis and osteoarthritis can also be aided by stretching exercises.

The increased oxygen intake from aerobic exercise aids the brain and the complexion. It helps to alleviate nervous irritability, depression, and anxiety. It also relieves tiredness and increases energy. Resistance to the common cold is enhanced, and sleep, weight loss, appetite control, and bowel regularity can be immeasurably improved. Cellular wastes are moved through the system for better elimination via the kidneys, bowels, and skin. Emotional health is also a by-product of regular exercise; a feeling of "centeredness" and well-being is often experienced by devotees of regular exercise. Exercise releases valuable endorphins, the brain's natural mood elevators, which contribute to feeling good and in control. Exercise may be the perfect prescription for those "menopause blues" that some women experience.

A Word of Caution: Avoid Overexercising

For women in adrenal burnout (see Chapter 2), exercising to exhaustion is counterproductive because it puts more stress on the adrenals. Too much exercise (over two hours of strenuous, nonstop activity on a daily basis) causes a halt in estrogen production—as in menopause—that can actually contribute to calcium loss in a very thin woman. Even when exercise is decreased and estrogen levels become normalized, a 20 percent bone loss can remain. If this cycle is repeated and the diet contains lots of calcium robbers such as coffee, sugar, and soda, premature bone thinning will set in before menopause begins. Just as with diet, balance should be the keynote in exercise.

Overexercise can also lead to hormonal imbalance. Increased loss of body fat brought on by strenuous exercise first causes progesterone levels to drop. Progesterone deficiency may ensue, and this leads to bone loss. The secondary consequence of increased fat loss is the depletion of estrogen stores, resulting in menstrual irregularities, including cessation of menstrual periods when body fat is 18 percent or lower. This situation is often evident in trained athletes such as bodybuilders, runners, and ballet dancers, who can turn their periods on and off with a three- to five-pound weight gain or loss. Women who were involved in athletics in their teens and twenties and who missed at least one-third of their regular menstrual periods might be wise to check out their current bone density. In older women, this exercise-induced hormonal imbalance may be confused with menopause.

Exercise can be particularly beneficial in helping Hot Times women guard against osteoporosis. Tufts University researchers suggest that regular walking may even reverse osteoporosis. In fact, most osteoporosis-prevention programs recommend a thirty- to forty-minute brisk walk at least four times a week. Exercise aids in calcium absorption, and helps to strengthen existing bone and stimulate the formation of new bone. Activities that are aerobic provide intermittent stress and strain, which actually stretches the bone and helps to maintain and build bone mass. The stress causes an electric current to go through the bone, triggering the calcification process—this is known as the piezoelectric effect. An added bonus for the Hot Times woman is that exercise can mobilize stored estrogen from the fatty tissue.

The Hot Times approach to exercise recommends a balanced aerobic, weight-bearing exercise program that may include brisk walking, hiking, biking, rowing, tennis and other racquet sports, weightlifting, and jumping rope—all of these activities will help to strengthen your bones and improve your overall health. (Swimming is not considered a weight-bearing exercise, because you're weightless in water.) Remember that weight-bearing exercise appears to be one vital element of the bone-building formula, because bones become stronger with physical stress. If they're not used, they lose calcium and become porous.

The Best Things in Life Are Free (or Almost)

The nice thing about most exercise is that it is available to everybody, at practically any time of the year, at little or no cost. An ideal, well-rounded exercise program should include certain kinds of exercises designed to meet the three basic physical fitness components: cardiovascular endurance, muscle strength, and flexibility. Choosing a variety of exercises that fit into these categories will ensure that the entire body gets a workout. While some of the exercises can be done at gyms and studios, they can also be done at home alone or with family and friends or your television set.

CARDIOVASCULAR EXERCISE

The cardiovascular activities known as aerobic exercises include swimming, bike riding, rowing, cross-country skiing, brisk walking, jogging, racquet sports, jumping rope, and aerobic dancing. What all of these activities have in common is that they require a sustained supply of oxygen for long periods of time. This conditions the heart and respiratory system, pumping oxygen to all parts of the body. For these exercises to be effective, you must sustain them, keeping up your heart rate for fifteen to thirty minutes. Cardiovascular exercises promote energy and endurance, and raise the level of the "happy hormones" in the bloodstream.

Rebounding for Health: Strengthening the Lymphatic System

Every second of every day, your body's cells are producing waste products and dying. Toxic substances, bacteria, cancer cells, and other disease-causing agents are moving throughout your body. While the circulatory system carries nutrients, oxygen, and hormones to our cells, the lymphatic system is the body's garbage disposal system. Its meshlike network of tiny vessels transports lymph (fluid) from around the cells through lymph nodes, where the waste products are filtered out, cancer cells are trapped, and bacteria are destroyed. As it moves through the intestinal organs, lymph also pulls fat out for transport to the liver. (Protein and carbohydrates are left behind to travel via blood to cells.) To keep this fluid moving, the system depends on the muscle action of your arms and legs.

When the lymphatic system isn't working properly, fluid accumulates around cells, which can result in up to fifteen pounds of excess weight. This fluid prevents nutrients from entering cells, depriving them of the nourishment they need to thrive. Fluid that accumulates in your legs binds to fat cells that become swollen; more fluid accumulates, and what results, many experts believe, is cellulite and varicose veins. Finally, bacteria, cancer cells, and toxins are left to damage cells and bring on ill health.

What does this have to do with exercise? A lot, it seems. Without an internal pump to move lymph along, the system depends on your muscle movement. And one of the best ways I've found to exercise the lymphatic system is the daily use of a rebounder, or mini-trampoline. No matter where you live, you can exercise the lymphatics by bouncing on a rebounder for five to twenty minutes a day.

The mini-trampoline has proved to be one of the most efficient, yet least harmful, forms of exercise. A high level of cardiovascular fitness and toning results from regular bouncing every day. The low-impact rebounding acts to gently move the waste materials in the lymph. Most people must start slowly and bounce for only five minutes at a time, then work up slowly until they are jumping for the suggested twenty-minute span. The light pressure on the thighs activates lymphatic drainage. Within two weeks, legs, buttocks, and ankles are better toned and fatty cellulite deposits begin to disappear.

The advantage of the mini-trampoline is its universality. It can be used by people of all ages, in all stages of life. Even handicapped people who cannot walk can sit on it or put their feet on it while someone else is bouncing and still receive lymphatic benefits. For a more strenuous workout, simply jump faster and lower. Bouncing is the exercise par excellence for all seasons and climates. The mini-trampoline is portable and versatile and requires no instruction. Every home should have one!

MUSCLE STRENGTH EXERCISES

For muscle endurance, the best choices include weight training, progressive resistance training on Nautilus machinery, push-ups, and sit-ups, at least twice a week. These exercises help tighten and tone the muscles, aiding weight loss because muscle tissue uses more calories than fat tissue. In addition to building muscle, these exercises build stronger bones, and strong, healthy bones are the best prevention for osteoporosis. Your local gym is probably your best resource to learn more about implementing a weight-training program by yourself or with a personal trainer. Don't be intimidated. I see women in their 70s and early 80s weight-training at the gym these days. These marvelous role models exude self-confidence and truly seem to enjoy what they're doing.

FLEXIBILITY

Flexibility exercises can be chosen from yoga, Pilates, tai chi, and special stretch and tone classes offered at many fitness and dance studios. Good for combating muscle and joint stiffness, these exercises make us bend, extend, and stretch. Flexibility exercises can help release stress and tension, besides alleviating physical tightness.

PUTTING IT ALL TOGETHER: YOUR WEEKLY WORKOUT PROGRAM

For women who have not been exercising on a regular basis, here is a sample weekly program that you can follow:

- Cardiovascular exercises: three days a week (for at least thirty minutes each day)
- Muscle-strength exercises: in alternation with cardiovascular exercises, three days a week (for at least thirty minutes each day)
- Flexibility exercises: daily (for at least twenty minutes)

My own schedule includes aerobic dancing three times a week for cardiovascular endurance, free weights three times a week, and a stretch routine every morning for flexibility.

HEALTH FOR ALL SEASONS

In the warm weather of spring or summer or in dry climates, drink water before exercising to replace fluids that will be lost in perspiration. The rule of thumb is a quart of water to a hundred pounds of body weight. Some fitness buffs feel best when they drink a glass of water on the hour to ensure sufficient hydration of body tissue. Some of the bottled mineral waters, such as Evian, are high in magnesium and potassium, which helps to balance body fluids.

In cold weather you must also drink a lot of water, because urine output triples in volume when the weather is cold. As in hot-temperature conditions, water can hydrate body tissue and will also help keep a steady body temperature. Remember to do your warm-up exercises indoors before exercising outdoors; this will acclimate your body to stressful cold temperatures.

For hot-weather fitness and health, cotton clothing is your best bet. Lightweight materials that can easily absorb perspiration and then dry quickly are advisable. Try to avoid antiperspirants, which block sweating, the body's natural cooling mechanism. This is particularly important for menopausal women who are experiencing hot flashes or night sweats.

In cold weather, clothing should be loose rather than tight-fitting. Choose the layered look, consisting of several layers of natural material. Insulation is provided by the warm air-filled spaces between the layers. Plastic fabrics or polyester should be avoided, because these fabrics do not allow the skin to breathe, a special concern for the prime-time woman. Do remember to keep your head and neck covered to protect body heat from escaping. Also, try to stay dry. Melting snow and rain create moisture, affecting clothing insulation. Water removes body heat at least twenty times faster than air.

There are combinations of cardiovascular, muscle-strength, and flexibility exercises that can be enjoyed seasonally. When the weather permits, it is distinctly more beneficial to exercise outside because of the added health bonus of sunlight. As previously discussed, the sun's rays aid in vitamin D production, which is critical to calcium absorption. The sun also provides stimulation to the optic nerve, which tonifies every gland in the body. Full-spectrum light from the sun also alleviates the cyclical mood-change syndrome known as seasonal affective disorder (SAD), a kind of depression that is characterized by lethargy and overeating. The light-hormone connection is well worth investigating if you have been suffering these problems, particularly in winter. If sunlight is not easily available, then you might want to purchase full-spectrum lights for application indoors. These lights are sold by Duro-Test Lighting (www.durotest.com).

The following is a list of the most suitable exercises for the different seasons and climates. If you have year-round access to health clubs, then include swimming and exercises for muscle strength as part of your total exercise plan.

- **Spring:** running, jogging, tennis, volleyball, badminton, stretching exercises or dance classes, roller skating
- **Summer:** walking/hiking, swimming, rowing, water skiing
- **Autumn:** brisk aerobic walking, bicycling, jumping rope, martial arts, stretching and toning exercises
- **Winter:** cross-country skiing, yoga, ice skating, tai chi, breath control
- **Wet climate:** walking, indoor sports, low-impact aerobics, stretching and toning exercises
- **Dry climate:** walking, low-impact aerobics, stretching and toning exercises

GAIN WITHOUT PAIN:
WARM-UPS AND COOL-DOWNS

A series of warm-up exercises for five to ten minutes is a good way to slowly ease into your exercise program. The purpose of these warm-ups is to limber muscles, to increase blood flow to all body parts, and to deepen your breathing for full exercise benefits. Light stretching, yoga postures, or calisthenics can prevent stiff muscles later on. Warming up the muscles is important, so as to avoid injury and to prevent muscle soreness, which could prevent you from continuing your exercise program. The same warm-up series of movements can be applied to cool-downs for five to ten minutes after the vigorous part of your exercise is completed. If you do not have time for both, the warm-ups are the more important.

The ultimate key to exercise is regularity. Many individuals make exercise a part of their daily regimen. Others exercise four days out of seven to keep the blood moving, muscles toned, and joints flexible. Whatever you decide to do, approach your program realistically and with joy. Exercise is a lifelong activity, so avoid crash programs, which can be painful and dangerous in the long run.

SEVEN

The Hot Times Diet

AFTER WORKING IN MY NUTRITIONAL PRACTICE WITH SO many women for so many years, I know a drastic change in eating habits can be overwhelming. With all the biological changes we undergo at menopause, this is not the time to make massive dietary changes all at once. The Hot Times Diet offers suggestions that you can implement step by step, food group by food group. When you limit or eliminate a food or beverage—such as coffee, for example—you can substitute a more healthful choice, such as roasted dandelion root tea. Try this on for size for at least a week before moving on to another healthy change. I know you can do it. I've seen thousands of women make improvements in their diet without changing their eating habits drastically.

The Hot Times Diet features the right fats, the right levels of complex carbohydrates, mineral-rich fruits and vegetables, and quality protein, all in moderation and balance. This diet is specifically designed for a woman's unique needs at menopause, as a key aid in protecting against heart disease, cancer, and osteoporosis, and improving overall health and well-being.

BEVERAGES

I have found that changing what you drink is a good first step toward better health. To begin, it is important to avoid coffee, regular tea, soda, and excessive amounts of alcohol because of their effects on calcium, magnesium, and the stress-fighting B vitamin levels in your body. Coffee and alcohol also exert a dehydrating effect on body tissue. Remember: alcohol is implicated in every negative health condition covered in this book (heart disease, low adrenals, diabetes, osteoporosis, and all the uncomfortable symptoms of menopause). However, limited amounts—2 to 4 ounces—may actually improve HDL cholesterol ratios and lower the incidence of cardiovascular disease.

The best beverage of all is clear, pure, noncarbonated water. Water helps rid the body of waste, keeps tissues moist and lubricated, and can help burn calories. A mere 5 percent loss of body moisture causes skin shrinkage and muscle weakness, just what we don't need at this time of life. I suggest drinking purified or bottled water from a reliable source or a water filter for your home.

Hot or cold herbal teas are good substitutes for sodas and coffee. In addition to containing no caffeine, many of these pleasant-tasting teas (such as rose hip, roasted dandelion root, and hibiscus) contain surprising amounts of vitamins and minerals.

HOT TIMES OILS

As previously discussed, oils provide essential fatty acids (EFAs), which are of prime importance at menopause, because they nourish dry skin, hair, and mucous membranes, as well as aiding in natural hormone production. Oil also helps in the transport of calcium into the soft tissues.

The Hot Times oils include flaxseed, rice bran, macadamia nut, coconut, and olive oils, all of which may be used year-round in baking and cooking (with the exception of flaxseed oil, which cannot be used in baking or cooking). These oils are included for their delicious nutty flavors, beneficial fatty acids, and stability at high temperatures (except flaxseed oil).

Unnatural fats—such as margarine, vegetable shortening, and processed and hydrogenated vegetable oils—should be avoided.

PROTEIN

Poultry, fish, beans and other legumes, selected soy proteins (tofu, tempeh, and miso), and lean red beef and lamb are good sources of readily available iron, zinc, and vitamin B_{12}, nutrients commonly deficient in a woman's diet, and are important elements of the Hot Times Diet. Omega-3–rich eggs are also a good source of minerals and may be enjoyed daily. Try to include vegetable protein sources such as beans, nuts, and seeds at least twice a week.

DAIRY PRODUCTS

Because of the magnesium-calcium interaction (see page 82), limit intake of high-calcium dairy products. I recommend two portions per day, maximum. No matter which dairy products you select, one portion equals 1 cup low-fat milk, 1 cup low-fat yogurt or low-fat cottage cheese, or 1 ounce hard cheese.

FRUITS AND VEGETABLES

Try to eat at least seven servings of fruits and vegetables per day. A vegetable serving is usually ½ cup cooked or 1 cup raw. Each serving contains 2 to 3 grams of fiber. I recommend fresh vegetables and fruits. Try to buy certified organic produce whenever possible. When unavailable, use frozen. Canned fruits and vegetables are the least desirable, because of the salt added in the processing.

Brightly colored orange and yellow vegetables—such as carrots, yams, squash, and sweet potatoes—are high in cancer-preventing beta-carotene. Green foods are magnesium- and vitamin A–rich. Bok choy, broccoli, kale, and sea vegetables are delicious sources of nondairy calcium. Remember, sea vegetables are also high in hard-to-find iron and trace minerals.

With the big interest in juicing these days, it is important to monitor intake. A glass of carrot juice generally contains four to five carrots without the dietary fiber, which slows down absorption of sugar. Carrots have a very high glycemic index, which means that in the form of juice, they can increase blood sugar levels very quickly. I recommend not drinking more than ¼ cup (2 fluid ounces) at one time.

Many women eat too much fruit in the mistaken belief that because it is natural it can be eaten without limits. Too much fruit, no matter what the source, can upset the delicate calcium balance in the system and increase triglyceride levels. If yeast problems are a concern, temporarily avoid all fruits for at least ten days or eat just one fruit a day. Serving portions for fruit can be found in Table 7-1.

COMPLEX CARBOHYDRATES

Up to two servings per day from this family of foods is recommended. Serving portions for complex carbohydrates can be found in Table 7-2. Fiber-rich grains like buckwheat, millet, and barley are particularly recommended for their high magnesium content. Whole unprocessed grains and legumes are good nonanimal protein and iron sources. Dried beans, peas, and lentils are tops in high fiber, with 4 to 8 grams per serving.

Table 7-1 Serving Portions for Fruit

Fruit	Serving portion
Apple	1 small (2-inch diameter)
Apple butter (sugar-free)	2 tablespoons
Apple juice or cider	⅓ cup
Applesauce (unsweetened)	½ cup
Apricots (dried and unsulfured)	4 halves
Apricots (fresh)	2 medium
Banana	One-half small
Berries: blackberries, blueberries, boysenberries loganberries, raspberries	½ cup
Cantaloupe	One-quarter (6-inch diameter)
Cherries	10 large
Dates	2
Figs (dried)	1 small
Figs (fresh)	1 large
Fruit cocktail (canned in juice)	½ cup
Fruit preserves and spreads	2 tablespoons (sugar-free)
Grape juice	¼ cup
Grapefruit	One-half small
Grapefruit juice	½ cup
Grapes	12
Honeydew melon	One-eighth (7-inch diameter)
Kiwi	1 medium
Mandarin oranges (canned)	½ cup
Mango	One-half small
Nectarine	1 small
Orange	1 small
Orange juice (any style)	½ cup
Papaya	½ cup
Peach	1 medium
Pear	1 small
Persimmon	1 medium
Pineapple	½ cup
Pineapple juice	⅓ cup
Plums	2 medium
Prune juice	¼ cup
Prunes	2 medium
Raisins	2 tablespoons
Strawberries	½ cup
Tangerine	1 large
Watermelon	1 cup

Adapted from A. L. Gittleman, *Supernutrition for Women* (New York: Bantam, 2004), with permission.

For women who are wheat- or gluten-sensitive, there are two grains in the menus that are great alternatives—amaranth and quinoa. These grains have a buttery, rich flavor. Amaranth, a tiny grain seed that is a fairly new addition to store shelves, was widely used by the Aztecs in Mexico hundreds of years ago and was revered as a magical, mystical grain. It is one of the highest-protein grains, at 20 percent. A ½-cup serving also has as much calcium as an 8-ounce glass of milk. Amaranth is a good source of lysine and methionine, essential amino acids lacking in almost all other grains. This unusual grain can be used alone as a cereal or added to the batter of breads and baked goods. Quinoa is as high as or higher in protein value than amaranth. Known as the "mother grain" of the Incas, quinoa is low in gluten but is an abundant source of the amino acids methionine and cystine, as well as lysine. Both of these grains are used as cereals and flour and are available without pesticides or sprays. Avoid all white-flour products.

Table 7-2 Serving Portions for Carbohydrates

Starchy Vegetables	
Food	**Serving**
Chestnuts, roasted	4 large or 6 small
Corn (cooked)	⅓ cup
Corn (on the cob)	1 (4 inches long)
Parsnips	1 small
Peas (fresh)	¼ cup
Potatoes, sweet or white	1 small
Potatoes, sweet or white (mashed)	½ cup
Pumpkin	⅓ cup
Rutabaga	1 small
Squash (winter types)	½ cup
Succotash	½ cup
Breads	
Bagel (spelt or sprouted grain)	½ small
Bread (spelt, sprouted wheat, rye, pumpernickel)	1 slice

Bun, hamburger or hot dog (sprouted grain)	One-half
Pita bread (sprouted-grain)	One-half (6-inch pocket)
Tortilla (sprouted-grain)	1

Cereals and Grains

Amaranth (cooked)	½ cup
Barley (cooked)	½ cup
Bran (unprocessed rice or wheat)	½ cup
Buckwheat groats (kasha, cooked)	½ cup
Cornmeal (cooked)	½ cup
Cream of Rice (cooked)	½ cup
Grits (cooked)	½ cup
Kamut (cooked)	½ cup
Kashi Heart to Heart Cereal	½ cup
Kashi Medley Cereal	½ cup
Millet (cooked)	½ cup
Oatmeal (steel-cut or old-fashioned, cooked)	½ cup
Popcorn (air-popped)	3 cups
Quinoa (cooked)	½ cup
Rice (brown, cooked)	⅓ cup
Rice (wild, cooked)	½ cup
Spelt (cooked)	½ cup
Uncle Sam Cereal	½ cup
Wheat germ	1 ounce or 3 tablespoons

Crispbreads and Crackers

Crackers (Bran-a-Crisp, FiberRich)	½ sheet
Crispbread, rye (Wasa)	½ sheet
Crispbread, Scandinavian-style (Finn-Crisp, Kavli)	½ sheet

Flours

Arrowroot	2 tablespoons
Buckwheat	3 tablespoons
Cornmeal	3 tablespoons
Garbanzo	3 tablespoons
Kuzu (root starch)	2 tablespoons
Rice	3 tablespoons
Soy	3 tablespoons

Legumes

Beans: black (dried, cooked), garbanzo (chickpeas), kidney, lima, navy, pinto	½ cup
Beans (baked, plain)	½ cup
Lentils (dried, cooked)	½ cup
Peas (dried, cooked)	½ cup

Pasta	
White, whole-grain, spelt (cooked)	½ cup

Adapted from A. L. Gittleman, *Supernutrition for Women* (New York: Bantam, 2004), with permission.

SEASONINGS

High sodium intake may be connected to high blood pressure, stroke, and heart and kidney disease. The first thing to do is cut all processed foods—such as chips, dips, and fast foods—out of the diet. Practically two-thirds of the sodium in the diet comes from these sources. Try to keep sodium intake at no more than 2000 to 3000 mg per day. I recommend using Morton Canning and Pickling Salt, which, unlike many varieties of sea salt on the market these days, is not contaminated with mercury. For additional flavoring ideas, try experimenting with garlic powder or onion powder, dill, parsley, cayenne, and dry mustard. Remember that the very hot spices, such as curries and chili peppers, encourage water retention.

NUTRITIONAL SUPPLEMENTATION

As a nutritionist, I believe—and I know my clients believe—that food is our best source of vitamins, minerals, enzymes, and amino acids for health. But because of hectic schedules, we can't always eat the way we know we should. To make matters worse, topsoil is now depleted of certain trace minerals—such as zinc, chromium, selenium, and magnesium—that are important for health. The stress of modern-day life, environmental pollution, and radiation all take their nutrient tolls on the twentieth-century body. Supplemental vitamins and minerals have become a necessity, not a luxury. It is no wonder that over 100 million Americans are supplementing their diets.

Here is an example of a comprehensive program that I typically will recommend to my clients:

- natural progesterone body cream (ProgestaKey): ¼ to ½ tea-spoon, once per a day
- OsteoKey: 3 capsules, two times a day
- magnesium: 1 capsule, once a day (separate from OsteoKey)
- vitamin E: 400 IU, 1 capsule, one to three times a day (for a total of 400–1200 IU)
- Female Multiple (copper-free): 2 capsules, three times a day
- Adrenal Formula (adrenal and stress support): 2 capsules, three times a day (for a total of 6 capsules)
- HCl digestive aide (hydrochloric acid and pepsin for diges-tive support): 1 to 3 capsules, three times a day (for a total of 3 to 9 capsules)
- Woman's Oil: 1 to 2 tablespoons per day
- StressCare: 2 tablets, two to three times a day (for a total of 4 to 6 tablets)
- MenoCare: 2 tablets, two times a day (for a total of 4 tablets)
- For my diabetic clients and those who crave sugar, I add 200 mcg chromium, two times per day. These supplements can be ordered directly from Uni Key Health Systems, my fulfill-ment center for all products, tests, and services, at 800-888-4353. Do remember that individual requirements may vary.

MINDFUL MEDICINE

Prescription drugs and over-the-counter medications can interfere with the digestion and absorption of key nutrients. For example, antibiotics and antacids affect calcium utilization. Diuretics eliminate potassium, zinc, and magnesium. Potassium is often prescribed with water pills, but zinc and magnesium are not—two minerals in short supply to begin with. Aspirin interferes with vitamin C and iron absorption, and can also magnify the effects of other medications, such as blood thinners. If you are taking prescription drugs, try to eat foods high in the vitamins that the medication depletes, or consider vitamin supplementation. Table 7-3 gives a listing of commonly prescribed drugs and their interactions with key nutrients.

It is helpful to know about drug interactions, so as to avoid reactions. Make sure that your primary physician is aware of every single prescription drug and over-the-counter medication you are taking. (In this age of medical specialists, it is common for people to see different physicians for different health concerns, getting medications from each doctor, none of whom may be aware of others' prescriptions.) Some drugs can cancel out the effect of others, magnify potency, or reduce their effects. You should know all potential side effects, whether your medicine should be taken with meals or without food, and the length of time you should be on it.

Table 7-3 Drug and Nutrient Interactions

Drug trade name	Major indication(s) for use	Effect on nutrient(s)
Achromycin V (tetracycline)	Gram-negative and gram-positive microorganisms	Reduces absorption of calcium, magnesium, and iron
Aldactazide	Hypertension, congestive heart failure, edema, diuretic action needed	Reduces potassium excretion
Aldactone	Hypertension, congestive heart failure, edema, diuretic action needed	Reduces potassium excretion
Apresoline	Hypertension	Depletes vitamin B_6
Aspirin	Minor pain	Causes deficiency in thiamine and vitamin C
Atromid-S	Cholesterol control	Reduces circulating vitamin K levels

Drug trade name	Major indication(s) for use	Effect on nutrient(s)
Azo Gantanol	Antibacterial, gram-negative and gram-positive urinary tract infection	Causes deficiency in folic add
Bentyl with phenobarbital	Functional gastrointestinal disorders, dizziness	Accelerates vitamin K metabolism
Brevicon	Oral contraception	Vitamin B_6 and C depletion
Bronkotabs	Bronchial asthma, bronchitis, emphysema	Accelerates vitamin K metabolism
Butazolidin	Rheumatoid arthritis and osteoarthritis, spondylitis	Causes deficiency in folic acid
Cantil with phenobarbital	Lower gastrointestinal, vitamin K distress, diarrhea, abdominal pain, cramping, irritable colon	Accelerates metabolism
Chardonna-2	Nervous indigestion, vitamin K gastritis, nausea, vomiting, spastic colon, flatulence	Accelerates metabolism
Colchicine	Chronic gouty arthritis	Decreased absorption of lactase, fat, sodium, potassium, and B_{12}
Cortisone tablets and suspension	Adrenocortical deficiency, allergic states, rheumatoid arthritis, dermatoses	Causes deficiency in vitamin B_6, zinc, potassium, and vitamin C; accelerates vitamin D metabolism
Demulen	Oral contraception	Depletes vitamins B_6 and C
Diethylstilbestrol	Menopause, senile vaginitis	Depletes vitamin B_6
Diupres	Hypertension	Increases magnesium and potassium excretion
Diuril	Hypertension	Increases magnesium and potassium excretion
Doriden	Insomnia	Causes deficiency in folic acid
Enovid E	Contraception	Depletes vitamins B_6 and C
Gantanol	Urinary tract, soft tissue, and respiratory infections	Causes deficiency in folic acid
Indocin	Rheumatoid arthritis, spondylitis, degenerative joint or hip disease, gout	Depletes vitamin C
Isordil with phenobarbital	Angina pectoris metabolism	Accelerates vitamin K
Lo/Ovral	Oral contraception	Depletes vitamin B_6
Mycifradin (neomycin)	Enterocolitis and diarrhea	Reduces lactase levels; causes vitamin K deficiency and malabsorption of vitamin B_{12} and folic acid

Drug trade name	Major indication(s) for use	Effect on nutrient(s)
Mycolog-II	Cutaneous candidiasis, infantile eczema	Reduces lactase levels; causes vitamin K deficiency and malabsorption of vitamin B_{12} and folic acid
Neo-Cortef	Contact and allergic dermatitis	Reduces lactase levels; causes vitamin K deficiency and malabsorption of vitamin B_{12} and folic acid
neomycin	Suppression of intestinal bacteria, diarrhea	Reduces lactase levels; causes vitamin K deficiency and malabsorption of vitamin B_{12} and folic acid
Neosporin	*Pseudomonas, Staphylococcus* bacteria	Reduces lactase levels; causes vitamin K deficiency and malabsorption of vitamin B_{12} and folic acid
Norinyl	Oral contraception, hypermenorrhea, rheumatoid arthritis	Depletes vitamins B_6 and C; increases vitamin B_6 requirement
OS-Cal	Osteoporosis	Depletes vitamin B_6
Phazyme	Gastrointestinal disturbances, aerophagia, dyspepsia, diverticulitis, spastic colitis	Accelerates vitamin K metabolism
Polysporin	Gram-negative and gram-positive microorganisms	Causes malabsorption of vitamins B_{12} and K and folic acid
Prednisone	Rheumatoid arthritis; joint pain, stiffness, swelling, and tenderness; asthma	Increases vitamin B_6 requirement; increases vitamin C excretion; causes zinc, potassium, and calcium deficiency
Premarin	Menopausal syndrome, senile vaginitis, pruritis	Causes folic acid deficiency; reduces vulvar calcium excretion
Pro-Banthine	Peptic ulcer, hypertrophic gastritis, pancreatitis, diverticulitis	Accelerates vitamin K metabolism
Ser Ap-Es	Hypertension	Depletes vitamin B_6
Sumycin (tetracycline)	Gram-negative and gram-positive microorganisms	Reduces absorption of calcium, magnesium, and iron
Tetracyn	Gram-negative and gram-positive microorganisms	Reduces absorption of calcium, magnesium, and iron

Even foods interact with drugs. Milk interferes with the absorption of certain antibiotics, such as tetracycline. Aged cheese, bananas, soy sauce, sour cream, and Chianti wine should not be taken with a monoamine oxydase (MAO) inhibitor, used to control high blood pressure. This combination can increase blood pressure to dangerously high levels, which could result in brain hemorrhage and death. Carbohydrates such as bread and crackers increase the time it takes for some over-the-counter pain relievers, like Tylenol, to take effect.

COOKING UTENSILS

It is best to avoid *all* aluminum-containing pots, pans, and foil, because aluminum hampers the body's utilization of calcium and phosphorus. High-quality stainless steel, cast iron, enamel-covered iron, Corning Wear, Pyrex, and other heat-resistant glass are preferable.

The real danger of aluminum comes from the aluminum hydroxides in many antacids, baking powder, and baking soda, and in the fluoride that is in aluminum foil. If you are going to freeze or refrigerate in aluminum foil, it is best to first wrap with waxed paper and then use the aluminum, so that none will leach into your food.

PUTTING IT ALL TOGETHER

Now you're prepared to enter into this new phase of your life, and to manage menopause the Hot Times way. Your transition to a diet low in processed foods and rich in nutrients, and your commitment to a consistent exercise regimen, will help ease you naturally into midlife. But you may be feeling a bit overwhelmed by so much information. What's the best way to get started?

Beginning on page 179 are the Hot Times Menus and Recipes, which will start your creative juices flowing. Just peruse the sections on breads, breakfast smoothies, beverages, appetizers and snacks, soups, salad dressings and salads, side dishes, entrees, and desserts, and you will see how inviting and sensuous Hot Times foods can really be. I have also included one-week diet samplers for each season, which showcase many year-round as well as seasonal recipes. These diet samplers are based on a Hot Times woman's unique nutritional needs. Along with the more contemporary dishes, you'll find recipes to help you prepare meals with an international flair. These recipes are simply a guideline and can be varied, depending on tastes. Feel free to interchange lunches and dinners based on your personal schedule. Most recipes serve 4 to 6 people, so you can serve these dishes at get-togethers or save the leftovers for freezing.

EIGHT

Hot Times Menus and Recipes

A NUTRITIOUS DIET THAT'S RICH IN VITAMINS AND MINER-
als and that includes the essential fatty acids is absolutely necessary
in maintaining physical and emotional well-being throughout
menopause. Perhaps you've already tried to make the transition to a
balanced diet, only to become confused by the multitude of vitamin-
and mineral-depleted products available in the marketplace. Anguish
no more! If you're preparing for your passage into midlife, and if
you're seeking to manage your menopause naturally, the Hot Times
menus will be your guide on the road to a healthier lifestyle.

Our eating patterns are partly dictated by what's available seasonally, as we seek to select the freshest food items available at the most
reasonable prices. For example, fresh raw fruits and vegetables are
more prevalent in our menus for summer, when they are readily available not only at the supermarket but also in our gardens. On the
other hand, more warming foods—such as soups, beans, cooked
grains, and root vegetables—tend to predominate in our winter fare.
As Perla Meyer, author of *The Seasonal Kitchen*, says, "Seasonal
cooking is catching freshness at its prime."

To assist you with your day-to-day meal planning, I have compiled one-week meal samplers. These will help you take advantage of the bounty of nutritious seasonal food items at hand in your local supermarket or natural foods store. Best of all, for each season, you will be introduced to a variety of healthful and delicious recipes that incorporate fresh produce, grains, legumes, dairy products, meats, fish, and vegetarian protein choices, as well as highly beneficial oils.

Now is the time to begin looking forward and feeling great. Eat up and enjoy!

HOT TIMES INGREDIENTS

Many recipes include Fat Flush Whey protein (available through 800-888-4353) and powdered stevia (a good brand is Stevia Plus), a natural low-glycemic sweetener available in health food stores and fine supermarkets. The Fat Flush Whey is derived from herds that are not treated with hormones. The whey is undenatured, unheated, rich in immune-boosting elements, and makes excellent smoothies.

You will also be introduced to a variety of exotic foods such as daikon and burdock, frequently used in Asian cooking, which contain healing properties for the female body. Daikon is a long white radish that assists digestion and metabolization of fats. Burdock, a medicinal root vegetable, is well respected for its blood-building and purifying properties. These ingredients, along with many others in the Hot Times recipes, are particularly high in minerals such as calcium, magnesium, and the essential fatty acids (EFAs).

Sesame seed paste, known as tahini, is an important ingredient because of its delightful taste and very high calcium content. Miso is a fermented soybean product that is a versatile cooking ingredient and is becoming quite popular in vegetarian cooking. It is especially noteworthy because it strengthens the blood and lymph and is a good source of enzymes, calcium, and iron. Tamari, an aged soy sauce, is another year-round item that is used in limited amounts as a flavorful alternative to salt, and aids in digestion. Tofu and tempeh are soy products that are nonanimal sources of good-quality protein and phytoestrogens. Kuzu is a thickening agent similar to arrowroot but is higher in minerals, particularly iron.

You will see many varieties of sea vegetables in the recipes. These vegetables have absorbed nutrients from the sea and are chock-full of hard-to-find trace minerals, as well as the more common calcium and iron (they have ten times more iron than spinach). Their nutritional qualities reach far beyond their rich mineral and vitamin content; most sea vegetables contain an element called sodium alginate that inhibits the absorption of radioactive and heavy-metal toxins. Sea vegetables are very versatile and can be used to flavor stews, spike soups, and enhance grains. The following list describes each vegetable and gives some suggestions for its preparation:

- **Agar** is a seaweed that is sold in flake form to be used in place of gelatin for thickening puddings, molds, and mousses. Agar is a high-fiber vegetable that is soothing to the digestive tract.

- **Arame** is one of the milder-tasting sea vegetables and would be a good one to use when introducing your taste buds to sea vegetables. Arame is high in iron, calcium, potassium, and vitamins A and B. It should be rinsed in cool water and soaked for ten to fifteen minutes. (Soaking will cause it to more than double in size.) It makes a tasty addition to salads, soups, brown rice, and vegetables. Both hijiki (discussed below) and arame can be sautéed for two to three minutes in oil.

- **Hijiki** tastes a bit like licorice and looks like tangled black strings. A half cup of cooked hijiki has almost the same calcium content as a half cup of milk. This vegetable should be rinsed in cold water and then soaked for twenty minutes. It can be added to soups or salads and is delicious sautéed with carrots and fresh ginger.

- **Kombu** is a kelp with a sweet/salty flavor that is an excellent source of minerals, such as magnesium, calcium, potassium, iron, and iodine. It can be toasted in the oven for snacks, added to beans to aid in digestion, or crumbled and sprinkled over fish, chicken, or rice dishes. Cut into strips, it can be added to soups.
- **Nori** (green laver or sea lettuce) is a nutty-tasting seaweed, high in the B vitamins and vitamin A. Nori comes in sheets that can be toasted and crumbled over vegetables, pasta, or fish. The sheets can also be used untoasted to wrap other foods.
- **Sea palm fronds** are another mineral-rich treasure. This variety of sea vegetation is my particular favorite, because when cooked, sea palm resembles green pasta ribbons. The taste is mild and it lends itself well to enhancing many dishes.
- **Wakame** is a delicately flavored dark green leaf. It is a rich source of vitamins A, B complex, and E. It should be rinsed in cold water and soaked for fifteen minutes. Add it to soups or dressings, or serve atop fish.

The above list provides just a sample of the wide variety of foods that are delicious, healthful, and satisfying. This chapter will provide you with suggestions for incorporating ingredients into your diet that will supply you with the nutrients your body needs. Once you have made the transition to the Hot Times approach, you should explore some of the foods we have discussed in this book and make eating them a part of your daily life. Armed with this information, you truly hold the key to managing your menopause naturally and effectively.

HOT TIMES WEEKLY MENUS

Here is a four-week sampling of a Hot Times menu plan that features satisfying and substantial meals that the whole family will enjoy year-round. The recipes that are noted within these sample menus are not only delicious and carb-conscious but they also will appeal to a variety of palates.

Spring

Monday

BREAKFAST:
Tropical Splendor Smoothie (page 209)
Sprouted-grain toast with unsweetened preserves

LUNCH:
Spring Minestrone (page 216)
Classic Hummus (page 216)
Fresh-cut vegetables

DINNER:
Baby spinach salad with fresh chives
Raspberry Vinaigrette (page 229)
Roasted chicken with tarragon and steamed asparagus

Tuesday

BREAKFAST:
Uncle Sam's Cereal
Low-fat plain yogurt with cinnamon
Fresh raspberries and blackberries with fresh mint

LUNCH:

Mixed green salad with radish and bean sprouts

Dressing of 2 tablespoons each almond oil and lemon juice and 2
teaspoons chives

Turkey cutlet sautéed in 1 tablespoon olive oil, with garlic, rosemary,
and lime

Steamed snow peas with fresh mint

DINNER:

Baked artichokes with garlic and lime juice

Sweet and Sour Tempeh (page 257)

Steamed brown rice with grated carrot and toasted sesame seeds

Wednesday

BREAKFAST:

Bahama Splash (page 211)

Poached eggs

Spelt toast with unsweetened preserves

LUNCH:

The Best Grilled Chicken Salad (page 233)

Calming Ginger Tea (page 211)

DINNER:

Chilled Red-Velvet Borscht (page 218)

Herb-Crusted Salmon Fillet (page 263)

Steamed baby mélange of asparagus tips, baby carrots, and green beans
drizzled with flaxseed oil

Thursday

BREAKFAST:

Kasha

Low-fat plain yogurt with cinnamon and 2 teaspoons honey

LUNCH:

Mixed Greens with Citrus Almond Vinaigrette (page 231)

Broiled scallops with fresh parsley, dill, and lime

Roasted sweet potato

DINNER:

Steamed baby artichokes with lemon or

Dilled Tofu Mustard (page 253)

Grilled chicken brushed with olive oil and lemon juice

Fresh Spinach Sauté (page 245)

Friday

BREAKFAST:

Scrambled eggs

Sunburst Muffins (page 195)

Grapefruit half

LUNCH:

Gazpacho Cooler (page 212)

Festive Greek Salad (page 230)

DINNER:

Curried Carrot Soup (page 217)

Mixed green salad with diced tomato, cucumber, and bell peppers

Dressing of 2 tablespoons almond oil, 2 tablespoons lemon juice, and
   fresh basil
Spelt Pasta with Mushroom Lentil Sauce (page 259)

Saturday

BREAKFAST:
Garden-Fresh Vegetable Frittata (page 204)
Stylish Drop Biscuits (page 198) with 2 teaspoons honey

LUNCH:
Broiled tuna steak with leeks and spring onions
Spaghetti Squash with Vegetables and Spring Herbs (page 246)

DINNER:
Just Peas If You Please (page 232)
Grilled baby lamb chops with fresh mint
Spinach-Stuffed Portobello Mushrooms (page 243)

Sunday

BREAKFAST:
Almond Sunrise Pancakes (page 199)
Honeydew and cantaloupe wedges
Cottage cheese

LUNCH:
Mixed baby greens salad
Asian Ginger Dressing (page 227)
Grilled natural beef patty with romaine and sliced plum tomatoes

DINNER:

Mixed greens with radish, sprouts, toasted sesame seeds, and chives

Dressing of 2 tablespoons rice bran oil, 1 tablespoon lemon juice, and oregano

Broiled shrimp with lemon, garlic, and fresh dill

Springtime Ratatouille (page 244)

Summer

Monday

BREAKFAST:

Fiery Tomato Veggie Frappé (page 210)

Sprouted-grain toast with flaxseed oil and cinnamon

LUNCH:

Chilled Lemon Miso Soup (page 218)

Fresh-cut vegetables

Light Miso Tahini Dressing (page 230)

Tofu Ceviche (page 260)

DINNER:

Red leaf lettuce with pear tomatoes, artichoke hearts, and carrot

Dressing of 2 tablespoons olive oil, 1 tablespoon lemon juice, and fresh basil

Blackened Red Snapper (page 262)

Steamed collard and mustard greens with apple cider vinegar

Tuesday

BREAKFAST:

Papaya and melon chunks

Kashi Medley

Cottage cheese with cardamom

LUNCH:

Chilled Celestial Summer Soup (page 219)

Grilled chicken breast with garlic and fresh basil

Marinated Vegetable Salad (page 235)

DINNER:

Sweet 'n' Sour Cucumber and Red Onion Salad (page 234)

Sassy Beef and Vegetable Kabobs (page 269)

Steamed kale with savory and apple cider vinegar

Roasted sweet potatoes

Wednesday

BREAKFAST:

Breakfast Crepes with Mixed Berry Purée (page 203)

Calming Ginger Tea (page 211)

LUNCH:

Tuna salad with celery, red onion, and chopped egg mixed with
Easy Homemade Mayonnaise (page 228)

Gazpacho Cooler (page 212)

DINNER:

Summer Confetti Salad (page 234)

Grilled Cornish game hens with lemon, garlic, and rosemary

Brown Rice with Parsley Nut Sauce (page 247)

Thursday

BREAKFAST:

Sliced nectarines and plums

Scrambled eggs

Spelt toast with natural peanut butter

LUNCH:

Chunky Spinach and Artichoke Dip (page 214)

Fresh-cut vegetables

Broiled mahi mahi with lime juice, cumin, and pine nuts

DINNER:

Cucumber Dill Soup (page 219)

Honey Lemon Chicken on the Grill (page 266)

Steamed yellow squash and zucchini with rice bran oil and thyme

Friday

BREAKFAST:

Omelet with spinach, red bell pepper, and cheddar cheese

Sprouted-grain toast with 2 teaspoons honey

LUNCH:

Chilled Asparagus with Roasted Bell Pepper Sauce (page 249)

Broiled lamb patty

Steamed carrots with fresh dill, drizzled with almond oil

DINNER:

Summertime Gazpacho (page 220)

Torn romaine leaves with cucumber, radish, and julienned carrot

Dressing of 2 tablespoons each lime juice and almond oil and 1
    tablespoon cilantro

Grilled sea bass fillets with toasted sesame oil, garlic, and tamari

Broccoli with Lemon Crumbs (page 248)

Saturday

BREAKFAST:

Morning Madness Smoothie (page 207)

Sprouted-grain toast with flaxseed oil and cinnamon

LUNCH:

Broiled scallops with garlic, ginger, cumin, and cilantro

Steamed chard with pumpkin seeds and apple cider vinegar

DINNER:

Thai Coleslaw (page 238)

Grilled veal chops

Steamed parsnips tossed with lemon juice and fresh dill

Grilled zucchini and beefsteak tomatoes with fresh basil

Sunday

BREAKFAST:

Banana French Toast with Lemon Honey Syrup (page 201)

Calming Ginger Tea (page 211)

LUNCH:

Warm spinach salad with cherry tomatoes and toasted pistachios (see
   inset Toasting Nuts on page 239)

Light Miso Tahini Dressing (page 230)

Broiled turkey patty with lettuce, tomato, and red onion

DINNER:

Baby greens with hearts of palm, plum tomatoes, and scallions

Dressing of 2 tablespoons lemon juice, 2 tablespoons olive oil, and 2
   teaspoons Dijon mustard

Broiled filet mignon with garlic and rosemary
Molded Vegetable Gel (page 248)

Fall

Monday

BREAKFAST:
Pumpkin Pie Smoothie (page 208)
Spelt toast with unsweetened preserves

LUNCH:
A Tomato Soup to Love (page 223)
Lovely Chicken Salad (page 237)

DINNER:
Grated beets with toasted sesame oil and apple cider vinegar
Simple Salmon Patties (page 264)
Steamed spinach with Walnut Miso Sauce (page 246) or garlic and
   lemon

Tuesday

BREAKFAST:
Oatmeal with Cranberries and Toasted Pecans (page 204)
Soft-cooked eggs
Calming Ginger Tea (page 211)

LUNCH:
Jerusalem artichoke salad with grated carrots, jicama, and parsley
   mixed with

Dressing of 2 tablespoons lemon juice, 2 tablespoons flaxseed oil, and
  garlic
Chicken breast sautéed in toasted sesame oil and tamari

DINNER:

Autumn Harvest Soup (page 222)
Hearty Hungarian Goulash (page 271)
Steamed spaghetti squash with garlic and flaxseed oil

Wednesday

BREAKFAST:

Apple slices sprinkled with milled flaxseed and cinnamon
Scrambled eggs
Sprouted-grain toast with macadamia nut butter

LUNCH:

Spinach, grated daikon radish, carrot, and onion salad mixed with
Asian Ginger Dressing (page 227)
Shrimp and bok choy sautéed in toasted sesame oil and garlic
Steamed brown rice with scallions and toasted almonds (page 239)

DINNER:

Mixed green salad with grated carrot, red bell pepper, and walnuts
Cranberry Lover's Salad Dressing (page 227)
Broiled halibut with lime, cumin, cilantro, and cayenne
Braised Brussels sprouts with pearl onions and nutmeg

Thursday

BREAKFAST:
Sliced bananas with cinnamon and raisins
Low-fat plain yogurt
Poached eggs

LUNCH:
Butternut Bisque (page 222)
"Pear-fect" Fall Salad (page 239)
The Greatest Graham Crackers (page 197)

DINNER:
Bean Florentine Soup (page 221)
Tempeh Chili (page 259)
Steamed okra with lemon and basil

Friday

BREAKFAST:
Frozen Baked Apple Smoothie (page 206)
Spelt toast with natural peanut butter

LUNCH:
Mixed green salad with jicama, tomatoes, and black olives mixed with
Mean Green Salad Dressing (page 229)
Broiled flounder with lemon, oregano, and garlic
Spaghetti Squash Pancakes (page 252)

DINNER:
Celery root with a splash of olive oil and lemon juice
Chicken Cacciatore (page 264)

Autumn Squash Soufflé (page 250)
Steamed green beans with lemon, thyme, and toasted hazelnuts
  (page 239)

Saturday

BREAKFAST:
Sliced pears sprinkled with milled flaxseed and cinnamon
Hard-boiled eggs

LUNCH:
Shrimp Niçoise Salad (page 236)
Calming Ginger Tea (page 211)

DINNER:
Thai Coleslaw (page 238)
Baked haddock fillet with tamari and grated ginger
Mashed sweet potatoes with cinnamon and coconut milk

Sunday

BREAKFAST:
Apricot and Almond Smoothie (page 205)
Sprouted-grain bagel half with cashew butter

LUNCH:
Broiled turkey cutlet with Sweet and Sour Sauce (page 258)
Potpourri of lightly steamed seasonal vegetables

DINNER:
Roasted rack of lamb with garlic and Dijon mustard
Quinoa "Risotto" with Caramelized Onions (page 251)
Aegean Green Beans (page 252)

Winter

Monday

BREAKFAST:

Omelet with tomato, onion, and green bell pepper

Low-fat plain yogurt with cinnamon

LUNCH:

Red leaf lettuce salad with

Raspberry Vinaigrette (page 229)

Bean Pâté (page 215)

Fresh-cut vegetables

Blue corn tortilla chips

DINNER:

Roast beef with wine, carrots, and onions

Wild and brown rice with shiitake mushrooms and garlic

Braised celery with lemon and anise seeds

Tuesday

BREAKFAST:

Sliced apples and pears sprinkled with cinnamon

Scrambled eggs

Spiced Cranberry Tea (page 212)

LUNCH:

Favorite Israeli Salad (page 242)

Classic Hummus (page 216) with sprouted whole-grain pita half

Tabbouleh Salad (page 240)

DINNER:

Wonderful Winter Stew (page 261)
Steamed Jerusalem artichoke hearts with garlic and lemon
Bok Choy in Ginger and Garlic Sauce (page 254)

Wednesday

BREAKFAST:

Cream of buckwheat
Grapefruit half
Soft-cooked eggs

LUNCH:

Orient Express Salad (page 241)
Mung Bean Dal (page 255)

DINNER:

Grandma's Chicken "Un-Noodle" Soup (page 226)
Tangy Holiday Chicken (page 267)
Surprising Sweet Potato Casserole (page 256)
Steamed green beans with lemon and cilantro

Thursday

BREAKFAST:

Apple Bread Pudding (page 200)
Low-fat plain yogurt with cinnamon
Poached eggs

LUNCH:

Spinach leaves with tomatoes, carrot, and toasted walnuts (page 239)
mixed with
Dressing of 2 tablespoons macadamia nut oil and 1 tablespoon
raspberry vinegar
Bountiful Bouillabaisse (page 225)

DINNER:

Moroccan Carrot Salad (page 241)
Middle Eastern Lamb Loaf (page 271)
Baked acorn squash with almond oil, ginger, and cinnamon
Steamed broccoli with garlic, cumin, cayenne, and lemon

Friday

BREAKFAST:

Oat bran sprinkled with milled flaxseed and cinnamon
Tangerine sections
Low-fat cottage cheese

LUNCH:

Brazilian Bean Dream (page 224)
Baba Ghanoush (page 213)
Fresh-cut vegetables

DINNER:

Wilted red cabbage salad with garlic and caraway seeds
Dressing of 2 tablespoons apple cider vinegar and 2 tablespoons olive
oil
Broiled swordfish steak with lemon, parsley, and rosemary
Hijiki Noodles (page 256)

Saturday

BREAKFAST:

Sliced bananas and grapes

Slice of cheddar cheese

Spelt toast with macadamia nut butter and milled flaxseed

LUNCH:

Vegetable broth

Roast beef slices wrapped in romaine leaves with Dijon mustard

Potpourri of steamed seasonal root vegetables with lemon

DINNER:

Green salad with diced tomato, cucumber, and bell peppers
    mixed with

Dressing of 2 tablespoons walnut oil, 2 tablespoons lemon juice, and
    fresh basil

Broiled salmon with lemon, garlic, cumin, ginger, and cayenne

Steamed kale with apple cider vinegar and garlic

Roasted sweet potatoes

Sunday

BREAKFAST:

Frittata with artichokes, red bell pepper, spinach, and feta

Spelt bagel half with 2 teaspoons honey

LUNCH:

Chicken salad with celery, red onion, dill, and parsley over romaine
    mixed with

Easy Homemade Mayonnaise (page 228)

Calming Ginger Tea (page 211)

DINNER:

Pot Roast with Sweet Potatoes and Vegetables (page 268)

Burdock Carrot Kimpira (page 254)

Roasted eggplant and tomatoes with

Warm Anchovy Sauce (page 249)

BREADS

· *Sunburst Muffins* ·

(MAKES 12 LARGE OR 36 MINIATURE)

1 cup milled flaxseed

½ cup ground walnuts

¾ cup vanilla Fat Flush Whey Protein (see page 176)

2 teaspoons aluminum-free baking powder

1 teaspoon baking soda

1½ teaspoons cinnamon

⅛ teaspoon ginger

¼ teaspoon salt

4 teaspoons macadamia nut oil

2 large eggs

¼ cup natural unheated honey

2 teaspoons vanilla extract

⅓ cup grated zucchini

⅓ cup grated carrot

¼ cup finely chopped Granny Smith apple or other baking apple

⅔ cup ricotta cheese

½ cup chopped walnuts (optional)

2 tablespoons raisins or finely chopped cranberries (optional)

Preheat oven to 350°F. Lightly coat the muffin cups with olive oil spray. In a small bowl, whisk together the flaxseed, walnuts, whey protein, baking powder, baking soda, cinnamon, ginger, and salt. Set aside.

In a large mixing bowl, mix together the macadamia nut oil, eggs, honey, vanilla, zucchini, carrot, apple, and ricotta. Fold the flaxseed mixture into the egg mixture. Fold in the chopped walnuts, if using, and the raisins, if using. Divide the batter evenly into the muffin cups. (Cups will be almost full.)

Bake 18 to 20 minutes or until a toothpick inserted into middle of a muffin comes out clean. Let cool; store in refrigerator. Serve with a drizzle of honey, if desired. These muffins freeze very well.

· Spelt Soda Bread ·

(SERVES 4)

2 cups spelt flour
¾ teaspoon baking soda
½ teaspoon salt
2 tablespoons milled flaxseed (optional)
6 tablespoons chilled butter
1 teaspoon caraway seeds
½ to ¾ cup almond milk (see Almond Milk recipe, page 197)
1 ounce tofu
1 tablespoon natural unheated honey
¼ to ½ cup garbanzo flour (for kneading)

· *Almond Milk* ·

1 cup water
½ cup ground almonds or almond meal

Bring 1 cup of water to a boil. Pour the water over the ground almonds and let steep for 10 minutes; blend. Pour through sieve
that has been placed over a small bowl.

Preheat the oven to 350°F. Mix together flour, baking soda, salt, and
flaxseed, if using. Cut in the chilled butter; stir in the caraway seeds.
In a small bowl, blend ½ to ¾ cup almond milk with the tofu and
honey. Mix together the wet and dry ingredients. Knead briefly, using
¼ to ½ cup garbanzo flour to make the dough smooth and elastic.
Shape the dough into a round loaf and place on a baking sheet that
has been lightly coated with olive oil. Cut a large cross in the top of
the loaf; spray lightly with olive oil. Bake for 50 minutes. Cut into 4
slices; serve warm.

VARIATIONS: Substitute raisins, sesame seeds, whole flaxseed, or
celery seeds for the caraway seeds.

· *The Greatest Graham Crackers* ·

(MAKES 20 CRACKERS)

1½ cups spelt flour
2 tablespoons toasted wheat germ
¼ teaspoon salt
½ teaspoon nonaluminum baking powder
¼ teaspoon cinnamon

3 tablespoons butter, melted

1 tablespoon molasses

2 to 4 tablespoons water

3 tablespoons natural unheated honey

Additional spelt flour, as needed

Preheat the oven to 350°F. In a medium bowl, sift together the spelt flour, wheat germ, salt, baking powder, and cinnamon. In a separate bowl, combine the melted butter, molasses, water, and honey. Combine with dry ingredients, using a fork.

Gather the dough together with your hands, being careful not to knead. The dough will be sticky. Place the dough on a spelt-floured surface and roll with a spelt-floured rolling pin to ⅛-inch thickness. Using a pizza cutter, cut the dough into rectangles (about 2½ inches by 2 inches, for a total of 20 crackers). Prick each cracker with a fork.

Place on a baking sheet lightly coated with olive oil; bake for about 15 minutes. Remove to a rack; let cool. Store in an airtight container.

· Stylish Drop Biscuits ·

(MAKES 12 LARGE BISCUITS)

2 cups spelt flour

1 teaspoon salt

2 ½ teaspoons nonaluminum baking powder

1 scoop vanilla Fat Flush Whey Protein (see page 176)

5 tablespoons chilled butter

1 cup water

Preheat the oven to 400°F. Mix the dry ingredients together. Cut the butter into the spelt flour mixture with a pastry cutter until it becomes the consistency of coarse cornmeal. Make a well in center of flour and add the water and any combination of suggested additions (below) as desired. Stir the dough for one minute. Drop onto an ungreased cookie sheet and bake 12 to 15 minutes.

SUGGESTED VARIATIONS:
- 4 tablespoons sautéed onions with the liquid
- 2 tablespoons finely chopped fresh parsley or chives
- ½ cup raisins, currants, or finely chopped cranberries
- 1 tablespoon date sugar added to flour mixture; dust with cinnamon before baking
- ¼ cup chopped nuts
- 2 tablespoons grated Parmesan cheese

BREAKFAST

· Almond Sunrise Pancakes ·

(MAKES 4 PANCAKES)

5 tablespoons coarsely ground almonds
1 scoop vanilla Fat Flush Whey Protein (see page 176)
½ teaspoon nonaluminum baking powder
1 egg, beaten
3 tablespoons Cranberry Quencher (page 210) or water
1 tablespoon pure maple syrup
2 tablespoons part-skim or whole-milk ricotta cheese
   (optional)
1 teaspoon vanilla extract
2 tablespoons macadamia nut or almond oil

SWEET CINNAMON BUTTER:

2 tablespoons butter, at room temperature

Dash cinnamon

Dash Stevia Plus (see page 176)

Mix almonds, whey protein, and baking powder in a small bowl. In a measuring cup, mix together the egg, Cranberry Quencher, maple syrup, ricotta cheese, vanilla, and macadamia nut oil. Combine well with the almond mixture.

Ladle ¼ cup of the batter onto a preheated frying pan or griddle that has been lightly coated with olive oil spray. Tilt the pan to allow the pancake to spread until it is about 5 inches wide. Cook over medium heat until the bottom of the pancake is golden brown and bubbles form on the top (about 3 minutes). Carefully flip the pancake; cook for another 2 to 3 minutes.

Freezes well. Serve with Sweet Cinnamon Butter. Drizzle with Lemon Honey Syrup (page 202) or ¼ cup pure maple syrup and 2 tablespoons flaxseed oil blended together.

To make the sweet cinnamon butter, whip together butter, cinnamon and stevia.

VARIATION: Stir 1 mashed banana into the batter.

· Apple Bread Pudding ·

(SERVES 2)

2 eggs

1 scoop vanilla Fat Flush Whey Protein (page 176)

¾ cup Cranberry Quencher (page 210) or water

1 Granny Smith apple, peeled, cored, and finely chopped

¾ teaspoon cinnamon

⅛ teaspoon cloves (optional)

⅛ teaspoon ground nutmeg (optional)
1 teaspoon Stevia Plus (see page 176)
1 tablespoon milled flaxseed
1 slice wheat-free, yeast-free spelt bread (French Meadow
   HealthSeed Spelt), torn into ½-inch pieces

Preheat the oven to 350°F. Fill a 9 x 13-inch pan with approximately ½ inch of water and place in the oven. Lightly coat a 3-cup ovenproof casserole dish with olive oil cooking spray.

In a medium bowl, beat the eggs lightly; set aside. In a separate bowl, whisk together the whey protein and Cranberry Quencher until smooth; whisk the mixture into the eggs. Stir in the remaining ingredients.

Pour the pudding mixture into the prepared casserole dish and place the casserole dish in the pan of heated water. Bake 45 to 55 minutes, or until a toothpick inserted into the center of the pudding comes out clean but is not completely dry. Let cool 5 to 10 minutes.

VARIATION: This dish is great served at any temperature. Try varying the fruit, using what is available seasonally, such as berries, pears, mangoes, peaches, nectarines, and bananas. It freezes and reheats well.

· Banana French Toast with Lemon Honey Syrup ·

(SERVES 6)

2 eggs
2 large ripe bananas
1 scoop vanilla Fat Flush Whey Protein (see page 176)
½ cup Cranberry Quencher (page 210) or water
½ teaspoon cinnamon
1 teaspoon vanilla extract

6 slices wheat-free, yeast-free spelt bread (French Meadow
   HealthSeed Spelt)
½ cup Lemon Honey Syrup (recipe below)

Blend the eggs, bananas, whey protein, Cranberry Quencher, cinnamon, and vanilla in a blender or food processor until smooth. Pour the mixture into a 9 x 13-inch pan. Place the bread in the banana mixture and let soak until the liquid is mostly absorbed, about 15 minutes, turning the bread occasionally.

Lightly coat a large heavy skillet with olive oil spray; heat over medium heat. Add the bread and cook until golden brown, about 3 to 4 minutes per side. Serve, passing warmed Lemon Honey Syrup separately. Freezes well.

· Lemon Honey Syrup ·

(MAKES ABOUT 1½ CUPS)

1½ cups natural unheated honey
½ cup water
¼ cup fresh lemon juice
½ teaspoon grated lemon zest

Combine all the ingredients in small a saucepan; cook over medium heat, stirring occasionally, until boiling. Boil the mixture until reduced by at least 25 percent. Serve warm. Store in an airtight container.

· Breakfast Crepes with Mixed Berry Purée ·

(MAKES ABOUT 4 CREPES)

CREPE BATTER:

2 eggs

1 scoop vanilla Fat Flush Whey Protein (see page 176)

½ teaspoon cinnamon

FILLING:

1 cup frozen berries

1 tablespoon water

1 tablespoon flaxseed oil

¼ teaspoon Stevia Plus or to taste (see page 176)

To make the crepe batter, blend the eggs, whey protein, and cinnamon together until smooth (the batter will be thin). For the filling, place the frozen berries in a small bowl and mix with the water; defrost briefly in the microwave to soften. Purée the softened berries, flaxseed oil, and stevia with a wand mixer or mini food processor; set aside.

Coat a crepe pan (or small frying pan) lightly with olive oil spray; place over medium heat. When the pan is hot (a drop of water will sizzle), pour a couple of tablespoons of batter into the pan, tilting quickly to cover the entire bottom with batter. Cook until the edges of the crepe begin to curl and turn golden. Flip carefully; cook briefly on the second side. Remove the crepe to a warmed plate. Continue making crepes until all the batter is used.

Place 2 to 3 tablespoons of berry purée along one edge of the crepe and roll up, arranging seam side down on plate. Pour remaining berry purée over the top of the rolled crepes.

· Oatmeal with Cranberries and Toasted Pecans ·

(SERVES 1)

1 cup water
⅛ teaspoon salt (optional)
½ cup old-fashioned oats
½ teaspoon Stevia Plus, or to taste (see page 176)
¼ cup fresh chopped cranberries, or other seasonally available
    fruit
1 tablespoon chopped toasted pecans

Combine the water and salt, if using, in a small saucepan; bring to a rolling boil. Stir in the oats and stevia, reduce the heat to medium, and cook 5 minutes, stirring occasionally. Cover, remove from the heat, and let stand 2 to 3 minutes. Pour the oatmeal into a serving bowl; top with the cranberries and pecans.

· Garden-Fresh Vegetable Frittata ·

(SERVES 4)

1 tablespoon olive oil
2 garlic cloves, crushed
½ cup chopped onion
¼ cup chopped Italian (flat) parsley
1 tablespoon chopped cilantro
¼ cup fresh diced asparagus, steamed
¼ cup cooked spinach, squeezed dry
¼ cup chopped plum tomatoes

6 eggs

½ cup shredded mozzarella cheese or other cheese

Salt, to taste (optional)

Cayenne, to taste

Preheat the broiler. Heat the oil in a medium ovenproof skillet with a lid. Sauté the garlic until softened. Add the onion, parsley, cilantro, asparagus, spinach, and tomatoes and sauté until tender-crisp. Remove the skillet from the heat; discard the garlic. In a medium bowl, blend together the eggs, cheese, salt, if using, and cayenne. Turn the heat to low; pour the egg mixture into the skillet, stirring well. Cover and cook about 3 minutes, or until the egg begins to come away from the sides of the pan. Place the skillet under the preheated broiler. Broil for an additional minute or until the frittata is set and lightly browned. Cut into 4 wedges and serve.

VARIATION: Other vegetables to try are artichokes, eggplant, mushrooms, bell pepper, and zucchini.

SMOOTHIES

· Apricot and Almond Smoothie ·

(SERVES 1)

1 scoop vanilla Fat Flush Whey Protein (see page 176)

½ cup fresh orange juice

1 tablespoon flaxseed oil

½ teaspoon Stevia Plus, or to taste (see page 176)

1 cup plain yogurt (low-fat or whole-milk)

1 cup fresh apricots, pitted, coarsely chopped, and frozen

2 tablespoons almond meal or ground almonds

1 tablespoon toasted wheat germ (optional)

1 tablespoon natural unheated honey (optional)

In a blender on high speed, combine all the ingredients until frothy. Continue blending on high speed for 2 to 3 minutes, or until thick and creamy. (If the mixture is too thick, stop the blender and stir with a wooden spoon; continue blending.) Makes 2 to 3 cups.

Hint: Freeze a portion of this smoothie for a yummy snack.

· Frozen Baked Apple Smoothie ·

Freeze the apple chunks the night before for fast and easy smoothie making in the morning.

(SERVES 1)

1 medium apple, peeled, cored, cut into chunks, and frozen

1 scoop vanilla Fat Flush Whey Protein (see page 176)

¼ teaspoon cinnamon, or to taste

¼ teaspoon nutmeg

Stevia Plus to taste (see page 176)

1 cup Cranberry Quencher (page 210)

1 tablespoon flaxseed oil

2 teaspoons fresh lemon or lime juice (can use up to 1 table-spoon)

When ready to make the smoothie, place all the ingredients in blender; blend on high speed about 3 minutes, or until thick and creamy.

· Cherry Berry Smoothie ·

(SERVES 1)

1 scoop vanilla Fat Flush Whey Protein (see page 176)
1 cup Cranberry Quencher (page 210)
1 tablespoon flaxseed oil
Stevia Plus, to taste (see page 176)
¾ cup frozen whole cherries, pitted
¼ cup frozen whole strawberries
1 cup crushed ice

In a blender on high speed, combine the whey protein, Cranberry Quencher, flaxseed oil, and stevia until frothy. Add the frozen fruit. Blend on high for 3 minutes, or until thick and creamy. Add the crushed ice; continue blending 2 to 3 minutes, or until desired thickness is reached. (If smoothie is too thick, stop the blender and mix with a wooden spoon; continue blending.)

HINT: Freeze a portion of this smoothie for a yummy snack.

· Morning Madness Smoothie ·

(SERVES 1)

4 ounces silken tofu
1 cup Cranberry Quencher (page 210)
1 tablespoon flaxseed oil
1 tablespoon milled flaxseed
1 tablespoon toasted wheat germ
¼ teaspoon cinnamon

Stevia Plus, to taste (see page 176)
½ cup frozen fresh pineapple
¼ cup frozen strawberries
¼ cup frozen blueberries
1 cup crushed ice

In a blender on high speed, combine the tofu, Cranberry Quencher, flaxseed oil, flaxseed, wheat germ, cinnamon, and stevia. Add the frozen fruit; continue blending for 2 to 3 minutes, or until thick and creamy. Add the crushed ice and continue blending about 3 minutes, or until desired thickness is reached.

· Pumpkin Pie Smoothie ·

(SERVES 1)

1 scoop vanilla Fat Flush Whey Protein (see page 176)
½ teaspoon cinnamon
¼ teaspoon ginger
⅛ teaspoon cloves
¾ teaspoon Stevia Plus, or to taste (see page 176)
1 tablespoon milled flaxseed
1 cup Cranberry Quencher (page 210)
½ cup unsweetened canned pumpkin
1 tablespoon flaxseed oil
1 cup crushed ice

In a blender, combine the whey protein, spices, stevia, and flaxseed. Add the Cranberry Quencher, pumpkin, and flaxseed oil. Continue blending for 2 to 3 minutes, or until thick and creamy. Add the crushed ice; blend about 3 minutes, or until desired thickness is reached.

VARIATION: Substitute 4 ounces silken tofu or ½ cup plain yogurt (low-fat or whole-milk) for the whey protein.

· *Tropical Splendor Smoothie* ·

(SERVES 1)

1 scoop vanilla Fat Flush Whey Protein (see page 176)
¾ cup coconut milk
1 tablespoon almond oil
1 tablespoon milled flaxseed
1 tablespoon chopped macadamia nuts
½ teaspoon vanilla extract
¼ teaspoon almond extract
Stevia Plus, to taste (see page 176)
½ cup frozen pineapple chunks
½ small banana
½ to 1 cup crushed ice

In a blender on high speed, combine the whey protein, coconut milk, almond oil, flaxseed, macadamia nuts, extracts, and stevia. Add the frozen pineapple chunks and banana; continue blending for 2 to 3 minutes, or until thick and creamy. Add the crushed ice; continue blending about 3 minutes, or until desired consistency is reached.

VARIATION: Substitute macadamia oil for almond oil.

· *Fiery Tomato Veggie Frappé* ·

(SERVES 1)

6 cherry tomatoes, frozen, or 1 medium tomato, quartered
2 tablespoons fresh lemon juice
1 scoop vanilla Fat Flush Whey Protein (see page 176)
2 teaspoons white horseradish
1 teaspoon low-sodium, wheat-free tamari sauce
1 tablespoon flaxseed oil
½ to 1 cup water (see Note)
¼ cup chopped, seeded cucumber
1 small carrot, shredded
1 scallion, chopped
⅛ teaspoon cayenne, or to taste
⅛ teaspoon celery seed
Dash salt

In a blender on high speed, combine all ingredients, blending for 2 to 3 minutes, or until thick and creamy.

NOTE: Start with ½ cup water. If a thinner smoothie is desired, use up to ½ cup additional water.

BEVERAGES

· *Cranberry Quencher* ·

(MAKES 4 SERVINGS)

4 ounces unsweetened cranberry juice or 1½ tablespoons
   unsweetened cranberry juice concentrate
3½ cups water

In a 32-ounce container, blend together the cranberry juice and water. Refrigerate. Sip throughout the day for a refreshing and healthy taste sensation.

· Calming Ginger Tea ·

(MAKES 2 SERVINGS)

3½ cups water
1-inch piece fresh ginger, sliced into thin rounds (about
    1 tablespoon)
6 cloves
1 cinnamon stick
Stevia Plus (see page 176) or natural unheated honey, to taste

Combine all the ingredients in a small pot. Bring to a boil and simmer for 10 minutes. Remove from the heat. Steep the tea for 10 minutes. (Tea will be cinnamon-colored.) Remove the ginger, cloves, and cinnamon stick. Drink hot or cold, served with a slice of lemon. Store the extra tea in an airtight container in the refrigerator.

· Bahama Splash ·

(MAKES ABOUT 1 QUART)

½ cup unsweetened cranberry juice
Juice of one lime
Juice of ½ grapefruit
3½ cups water
Handful of ice cubes

Stevia Plus to taste (see page 176)
1 tablespoon chopped fresh mint (optional)
Fresh mint sprigs, for garnish

Place all the ingredients (except mint) in a blender and blend until smooth. Stir in the chopped mint, if using. Pour into tall glasses; garnish with the mint sprigs.

· Spiced Cranberry Tea ·

(SERVES 1)

1 cup Cranberry Quencher (page 210)
2 tablespoons unsweetened fresh orange juice
1 tablespoon fresh lemon juice
Pinch ground ginger
Pinch ground cloves (optional)
1 cinnamon stick

Place all the ingredients in a small saucepan; stir. Heat to a boil; reduce heat and simmer for 5 to 10 minutes. Pour the tea into a large mug and serve with the cinnamon stick.

· Gazpacho Cooler ·

(SERVES 4)

1 medium cucumber, peeled and diced
2 tablespoons chopped celery
1 tablespoon chopped red onion

2 teaspoons apple cider vinegar
2 tablespoons fresh lemon juice
2 tablespoons fresh lime juice
Salt, to taste
Cayenne, to taste
4 cups low-sodium vegetable juice (see Note)
Crushed ice
4 small celery stalks, for garnish

In a blender on high speed, lightly purée the cucumber, celery, onion, vinegar, lemon and lime juices, salt, and cayenne. Combine the vegetable juice and the cucumber mixture in a large pitcher. Chill for 1 hour. Pour into tall glasses over crushed ice. Serve with celery stalk stirrers.

NOTE: Muir Glen 100% Vegetable Juice and Knudsen Very Veggie Organic Juice are good brands.

APPETIZERS AND SNACKS

· Baba Ghanoush ·

(SERVES 4)

1 medium eggplant
1 onion, sliced into thin half rings
1 tablespoon olive oil
5 garlic cloves, mashed
¼ teaspoon salt
¼ cup tahini

1 teaspoon turmeric
1 tablespoon cumin
1 teaspoon cayenne, or to taste
3 tablespoons fresh lemon juice
Chopped tomatoes
Chopped black olives
Olive oil or flaxseed oil (optional)
Fresh-cut vegetables, for serving

Roast the eggplant over an open flame or in a 450°F oven (prick skin) until skin darkens and collapses; let cool. Remove the skin and chop the flesh. Sauté the onion in the olive oil until lightly browned. Add the garlic and salt; sauté for 1 minute. Add the eggplant and continue sautéing for about 3 minutes or until the liquid is reduced. Add the tahini, turmeric, cumin, cayenne, and lemon juice; mashing well. Taste and adjust seasonings. Top with the tomatoes and olives. When ready to serve, drizzle with olive oil or flaxseed oil, if desired. Serve with fresh-cut vegetables.

· Chunky Spinach and Artichoke Dip ·

(MAKES 1½ CUPS)

1 (14-ounce) can artichokes, drained, rinsed, and coarsely
   chopped
2 (10-ounce) packages frozen spinach, defrosted and
   squeezed dry
⅓ cup finely chopped red bell pepper
1 (3-ounce) can water chestnuts, coarsely chopped
1 tablespoon Easy Homemade Mayonnaise (page 228) or
   Spectrum Naturals Organic Mayonnaise

1 tablespoon fresh lemon juice
¼ teaspoon dried dillweed
2 to 3 roasted garlic cloves, mashed
Cayenne, to taste

Combine all the ingredients in small bowl; mix well. Cover and chill.

VARIATION: For a cheesy taste, add 2 tablespoons freshly grated Parmesan cheese.

· Bean Pâté ·

(MAKES 4 CUPS)

4 cups aduki beans, cooked and drained
1 tablespoon light miso
¼ teaspoon cayenne
2 tablespoons rice vinegar
2 tablespoons extra-virgin olive oil
1 garlic clove, minced
1 teaspoon dried thyme
1 teaspoon dried oregano

Blend all the ingredients in a blender or food processor. Serve with tortillas or crackers.

· Classic Hummus ·

(MAKES ABOUT 1¼ CUPS)

1 (15-ounce) can chickpeas, drained (reserve 1 tablespoon
   liquid)
4 garlic cloves, minced, or more if desired
Juice of 1 lemon, plus additional for drizzling
1 tablespoon tahini
2 teaspoons olive oil, plus additional for drizzling
Cayenne, to taste (optional)

Coarsely purée the chickpeas, garlic, lemon juice, tahini, and olive oil
in a blender or mini food processor. Season with cayenne to taste. If
a smoother consistency is desired, slowly stir in the reserved tablespoon of chickpea liquid, mixing well. Drizzle with the additional
olive oil and lemon juice; sprinkle with cayenne if desired.

SOUPS

· Spring Minestrone ·

(SERVES 6)

1 onion, sliced
1 teaspoon olive oil
6 cups water
2 celery stalks, chopped
3 medium carrots, cut into rounds
1 cup broccoli florets
1 medium sweet potato, cut into cubes

1 cup sliced mushrooms

1 cup green bean pieces, 1 inch long

1 cup sweet peas

1 strip kombu (sea vegetable) (optional)

1 teaspoon chopped marjoram

1 teaspoon chopped thyme

2 tablespoons chopped parsley

¼ teaspoon salt (optional)

Sauté the onion in the oil over low heat until translucent. Add the water and bring to a boil. Add all the other vegetables and herbs and stir for 1 minute. Cover and simmer for 20 to 30 minutes. Remove kombu. Season with salt, if desired. The soup can be served either hot or cold.

· Curried Carrot Soup ·

(SERVES 6)

2 teaspoons extra-virgin olive oil

1 onion, coarsely chopped

5 medium carrots, coarsely chopped

1 teaspoon thyme

1 tablespoon curry powder

6 cups chicken stock or vegetable stock

2 tablespoons fresh lemon juice

1½ tablespoons light miso

6 parsley sprigs, for garnish

Heat the oil in a saucepan and gently sauté the onion until translucent. Add the carrots and thyme. Stir in the curry powder and sauté a few minutes longer. Add the stock and lemon juice. Simmer for 30 to 40 minutes. Blend with the miso and garnish with the parsley sprigs.

· Chilled Red-Velvet Borscht ·

(SERVES 6)

6 large whole beets, scrubbed and rinsed
3 large whole carrots, scrubbed and rinsed
8 cups water
1½ tablespoons light miso

Place the beets and carrots in the water and bring to a boil. When the beets and carrots are soft, remove from the water and cut into pieces. Place the vegetables and liquid in a blender or food processor and add the miso. Blend until smooth, then chill.

· Chilled Lemon Miso Soup ·

(SERVES 6)

6½ cups chicken stock or fish stock
2⅛ tablespoons light miso
3 tablespoons fresh lemon juice
1 medium carrot, cut into flowers
3 scallions, finely chopped
6 parsley sprigs, for garnish

Heat the stock in a soup pot. Take out 1 cup and dissolve the miso in it. Remove the pot from the heat and add the miso, lemon juice, carrot flowers, and scallions. Chill and serve garnished with the parsley sprigs.

· Chilled Celestial Summer Soup ·

(SERVES 6)

1 tablespoon sesame oil
3 leeks, chopped
2 garlic cloves, minced
3 tomatoes, peeled and chopped
5 cups vegetable stock
1 teaspoon chopped basil
1 tablespoon light miso
6 fresh basil sprigs, for garnish

Heat the oil in a soup pot. Sauté the leeks and garlic until the leeks are translucent. Add the tomatoes and sauté a few minutes longer. Add the stock and simmer 5 minutes. Purée in a blender or food processor with the basil and miso. Serve chilled, garnished with the basil sprigs.

· Cucumber Dill Soup ·

(SERVES 6)

6 cucumbers, peeled and cut into 1½-inch slices
4 cups water
3 tablespoons minced dillweed
2 tablespoons grated lemon zest
1 tablespoon light miso
Juice of 1 lemon
6 dillweed sprigs, for garnish
6 lemon slices, for garnish

Place the cucumbers in a soup pot with the water, dillweed, and lemon zest. Cover and simmer until the cucumbers are soft. Purée in a blender or food processor with the miso and lemon juice. Serve chilled, garnished with the dillweed sprigs and lemon slices.

· Summertime Gazpacho ·

If possible, refrigerate the gazpacho overnight to let the flavors develop.

(SERVES 12)

1 bunch celery, trimmed and chopped
6 Kirby cucumbers, chopped, or 3 large, peeled
3 red bell peppers, chopped
2 green bell peppers, chopped
2 yellow bell peppers, chopped
1 small red onion, chopped
4 large ripe tomatoes, chopped
1 (28-ounce) can diced tomatoes (Muir Glen)
1 (28-ounce) can tomato purée (Muir Glen)
Juice of 6 lemons (plus additional for serving—optional)
Juice of 4 limes (plus additional for serving—optional)
1 bunch Italian (flat) parsley, minced
¼ cup apple cider vinegar, or to taste (plus additional for
    serving—optional)
Cayenne, to taste

Combine the chopped celery, cucumbers, peppers, onion, and fresh tomatoes in a large bowl. Stir in the diced canned tomatoes and canned tomato purée. Purée one-third to one-half the mixture (in batches) in a blender or food processor; blend until the gazpacho reaches the desired consistency. Return the blended portion to the remaining gazpacho in the bowl; stir in the lemon and lime juices, parsley (reserve some for garnish), apple cider vinegar, and cayenne. Chill. Before serving, enhance the flavor by adding more lemon and lime juices, apple cider vinegar, and cayenne, if desired. Serve cold, sprinkle with the reserved minced parsley.

· Bean Florentine Soup ·

(SERVES 6)

2 cups dried navy beans
1 strip kombu (sea vegetable) (optional)
8 cups water
½ cup chopped celery
½ cup chopped onion
1 tablespoon chopped oregano
1 tablespoon chopped basil
1 teaspoon minced garlic
2 cups chopped spinach
¼ teaspoon low-sodium, wheat-free tamari

Place the beans and kombu, if using, in a soup pot with the water. Cover and cook about 1½ hours, until soft and creamy. Add the celery, onion, oregano, basil, and garlic. Cook 30 minutes longer. Add the spinach and cook 5 more minutes. Add the tamari and serve.

· Butternut Bisque ·

(SERVES 6)

4 cups water
1 large butternut squash, peeled and cubed
¼ teaspoon salt (optional)
¼ teaspoon cumin
¼ teaspoon coriander
¼ teaspoon grated ginger
¼ teaspoon garlic powder
6 parsley sprigs, for garnish
12 toasted almonds, for garnish
6 heaping tablespoons nonfat plain yogurt

Place the water and squash in a soup pot. Cover and simmer for 5 minutes. Add the salt, if using, cumin, coriander, ginger, and garlic powder. Continue simmering for 15 minutes. Purée in a blender or food processor. Serve garnished with parsley sprigs, almonds, and dollops of yogurt.

· Autumn Harvest Soup ·

(SERVES 6)

3 tablespoons sesame oil
1 cup chopped onions
1 cup chopped mushrooms
3 tablespoons dry sherry
8 cups vegetable stock
½ cup barley

½ teaspoon salt (optional)

6 parsley sprigs, for garnish

Heat the oil in a soup pot and sauté the onions until translucent. Add the mushrooms and sherry. Sauté a few minutes longer. Add the stock, barley, and salt, if using. Simmer for 45 minutes. Garnish with the parsley sprigs.

· A Tomato Soup to Love ·

(SERVES 4)

1 small onion, chopped

4 garlic cloves, minced

1 cup chopped celery

1 small carrot, grated

5½ cups homemade chicken stock or beef stock (or broth)

4 cups diced fresh tomatoes (about 5 to 6 large) or 2 (28-ounce) cans organic diced tomatoes (Muir Glen)

2 tablespoons chopped parsley

1 bay leaf

¼ cup chopped basil

Salt, to taste

Cayenne, to taste

Additional herbs and spices, as desired

Coat a 4½-quart pot or small Dutch oven with olive oil spray. Sauté the onion, garlic, celery, and carrot until softened and lightly browned; add the stock. Add the tomatoes, parsley, bay leaf, basil, salt, and cayenne. Add other herbs and spices as desired. Cover and simmer for 30 minutes to 1 hour, being careful the soup does not spill over. Remove the bay leaf and serve.

VARIATIONS: For Cream of Tomato Soup, mix 2 tablespoons unfla-
vored whey protein with 1 cup stock, broth, or water. Process in a
blender or food processor until thoroughly combined. Before serving,
gradually stir the whey mixture into the soup; warm through. Remove
the bay leaf and serve. For a complete meal, stir 2 cups cooked
shrimp or chicken into the soup for the last 5 minutes of cooking. Remove the bay leaf. Serve hot.

· *Brazilian Bean Dream* ·

(SERVES 6)

1 onion, chopped
2 garlic cloves, minced
2 tablespoons olive oil
1 cup dry black beans
2½ cups chicken stock
½ cup dry red wine
1 bay leaf
¼ teaspoon cayenne
2 celery stalks, chopped
1 tomato, chopped
¼ teaspoon salt (optional)

In a large heavy pot, sauté the onion and garlic in the oil. Add the
beans, stock, wine, bay leaf, and cayenne. Bring to a boil and simmer
2 minutes. Cover and let sit 1 hour. Add the celery and tomato. Simmer for 2 hours, or until beans are tender. Add salt, if using. Remove
1 cup of beans, mash, and return to the pot. Remove the bay leaf.

· *Bountiful Bouillabaisse* ·

(SERVES 6)

¼ cup peanut oil
1 onion, sliced
2 leeks, chopped
1 carrot, chopped
1 stalk celery, chopped
1 pound cod fillet, cut into 2-inch pieces
4 pound rockfish fillet, cut into 2-inch pieces
2 garlic cloves, chopped
1 bay leaf
1 teaspoon fennel seed
2 tablespoons Pernod (optional)
½ cup dry white wine
2 medium tomatoes, sliced
½ teaspoon salt (optional)
Cayenne, to taste
2 tablespoons minced parsley, for garnish

In a heavy pan, heat the oil and sauté the onion, leeks, carrot, and celery. Add the fish, garlic, bay leaf, and fennel seed. Sauté a few minutes more. Add the Pernod, if using, wine, and tomatoes. Add water to cover the fish and vegetables. Simmer for 30 minutes. Remove the bay leaf. Add the salt, if using, and cayenne, and serve garnished with the minced parsley.

· Grandma's Chicken "Un-Noodle" Soup ·

(SERVES 8)

12 cups homemade chicken stock or low-fat, low-sodium
   broth
½ teaspoon salt (optional)
1 bay leaf
4 garlic cloves, crushed
½ teaspoon cumin
1 cup chopped celery
1 cup chopped onion
3 cups diced cooked chicken
2 cups cooked spaghetti squash
1 tablespoon minced chives or finely chopped scallions, for
   garnish

In a large saucepan or Dutch oven, combine the stock, salt, if using, bay leaf, garlic, and cumin. Bring to a boil; add the celery and onion. Cover and reduce the heat to medium; simmer for 15 minutes. Stir in the chicken and spaghetti squash. Cook an additional 15 minutes, or until the soup is thoroughly heated. Remove the bay leaf. Garnish with the chives.

VARIATIONS: If a thicker soup is desired, mix 2 teaspoons arrow-root powder into ½ cup broth; stir into the soup. After the soup has simmered for 15 minutes, stir in 1 small cooked mashed sweet potato. Cook an additional 5 minutes; stir in the chicken and spaghetti squash. Or instead of spaghetti squash "noodles," you may use 3 or 4 medium zucchini, peeled and shredded lengthwise. (Avoid using seeded portion.) Stir in zucchini "noodles" for the last 5 minutes of cooking.

SALAD DRESSINGS AND SALADS

· Asian Ginger Dressing ·

(MAKES ABOUT 8 SERVINGS)

3 garlic cloves, minced
2 tablespoons minced ginger
½ cup rice bran oil or flaxseed oil
¼ cup sesame oil
⅓ cup rice vinegar or apple cider vinegar
½ cup low-sodium, wheat-free tamari
½ teaspoon Stevia Plus (see page 176)
¼ cup water

Process all the ingredients in a blender or mini food processor. Cover and refrigerate.

· Cranberry Lover's Salad Dressing ·

(MAKES 4 SERVINGS)

½ cup flaxseed oil
2 tablespoons apple cider vinegar
½ cup unsweetened cranberry juice (see Note)
¼ teaspoon dry mustard
¼ teaspoon minced garlic
¼ teaspoon ginger or turmeric
¼ teaspoon cinnamon

Juice of ½ lime, or to taste

½ teaspoon Stevia Plus or to taste (page 176),

Process all the ingredients in a blender or mini food processor. Cover and refrigerate.

NOTE: You can substitute 1 tablespoon unsweetened cranberry juice concentrate mixed with 3½ ounces water for the unsweetened cranberry juice.

· *Easy Homemade Mayonnaise* ·

(MAKES 1 CUP)

1 egg

½ teaspoon dry mustard, or to taste

Dash cayenne

½ teaspoon garlic powder, or to taste

½ cup extra-virgin olive oil

1 tablespoon fresh lemon juice

Combine the egg, mustard, cayenne, and garlic powder in a blender. Drizzle in the olive oil slowly, while continuing to blend, until the mixture becomes very thick. Scrape down the sides of the blender. Add the lemon juice; pulse briefly to mix. Cover and refrigerate.

VARIATION: Try replacing olive oil with almond, walnut, or macadamia oil for a mild nutty flavor.

· Mean Green Salad Dressing ·

Make this salad dressing and refrigerate at least two hours
before you plan to use it so it will be nice and "creamy."

(MAKES ABOUT 2 CUPS)

¾ cup water

½ scoop vanilla Fat Flush Whey Protein (see page 176)

1 medium scallion, coarsely chopped

1 garlic clove

3 tablespoons chopped parsley

⅛ teaspoon salt

1 tablespoon umeboshi plum paste (available in many health
  food stores)

⅓ cup flaxseed oil

3 tablespoons tahini

3 ounces firm tofu

¼ teaspoon cayenne, or to taste

Place the water in a blender. Add the whey protein and pulse briefly
to mix. Add the remaining ingredients and blend until smooth. Let
stand in the refrigerator for at least 2 hours to thicken.

· Raspberry Vinaigrette ·

Delicious on leafy salads.

(MAKES ABOUT 1 CUP, OR 8 SERVINGS)

½ cup raspberries, fresh or frozen

¼ to ½ cup water

2 tablespoons rice bran oil or flaxseed oil

1½ tablespoons apple cider vinegar
Dash Stevia Plus (see page 176)

Process all the ingredients in a blender or mini food processor; strain if seeds are not desired. Refrigerate in an airtight container.

· Light Miso Tahini Dressing ·

This dressing goes well on steamed greens, broccoli, and cauliflower.

(SERVES 6)

3 tablespoons tahini
1½ tablespoons light miso
1½ tablespoons brown rice vinegar
¼ teaspoon barley malt
½ teaspoon toasted sesame oil
¼ cup water, or more

Blend all the ingredients well. Add more water for a more liquid dressing, if desired.

· Festive Greek Salad ·

(SERVES 4)

8 cups torn romaine lettuce
1 cucumber, peeled, halved, and sliced
1 green bell pepper, seeded and cut into rings
½ small red onion, thinly sliced and separated into rings
4 plum tomatoes, cut into wedges

1 garlic clove, minced

⅓ cup extra-virgin olive oil

Juice of ½ lemon

½ teaspoon dried oregano, or to taste, plus additional for
   garnish

Salt, to taste

½ cup black olives, halved

½ cup crumbled feta cheese

8 anchovy fillets (optional)

¼ cup chopped Italian (flat) parsley

In a large salad bowl, toss together the romaine, cucumber, green pepper, onion, and tomatoes. In a blender, mini food processor, or jar with a tight-fitting lid, combine the garlic, olive oil, lemon juice, oregano, and salt, blending well. Pour the dressing over the salad, tossing well. Top with the black olives, feta cheese, and anchovies, if using. Sprinkle with the chopped parsley and additional oregano.

Variation: For a complete meal, add 1 pound grilled chicken breast, cut into strips.

· *Mixed Greens with Citrus Almond Vinaigrette* ·

(SERVES 4)

ALMOND VINAIGRETTE:

2 tablespoons fresh orange juice

2 tablespoons fresh lemon juice

2 teaspoons apple cider vinegar

2 teaspoons coarse-grained Dijon mustard

2 garlic cloves, minced (optional)

½ teaspoon Stevia Plus, or to taste (see page 176)

1 teaspoon grated orange zest
1 teaspoon grated lemon zest
½ cup almond oil

SALAD:
8 cups assorted torn salad greens (spinach, baby greens, red
   leaf lettuce, etc.)
¼ cup diced red bell pepper, for garnish
¼ cup diced carrot, for garnish
2 tablespoons toasted slivered almonds, for garnish

To make the dressing, combine the orange and lemon juices, vinegar, mustard, garlic, stevia, and zests in a blender or mini food processor. Slowly add the almond oil, blending until the dressing thickens. (Makes about ¾ cup.) Arrange the salad greens on a plate. Drizzle the dressing over the greens; garnish with the diced bell pepper, carrot, and toasted slivered almonds.

· Just Peas If You Please ·

(SERVES 4)

½ pound fresh peas (snow, sugar snap, shell, etc.)
Salt, to taste
2 teaspoons butter
2 teaspoons chopped mint
1 tablespoon chopped Italian (flat) parsley
1 tablespoon chopped cilantro
4 cups mixed baby greens
Fresh mint sprigs, for garnish

Remove the strings from the snow and sugar snap peas; shuck the fresh peas. In a medium pan of boiling salted water, boil the peas only until tender, 1 to 2 minutes. Drain well; return the peas to the pan. Stir in the salt, butter, and chopped herbs; chill. Arrange the baby greens on plates; top with the peas and garnish with the mint sprigs.

· The Best Grilled Chicken Salad ·

(SERVES 4)

4 cups torn fresh spinach leaves
2 cups torn green or red leaf lettuce, romaine, or baby greens
2 tablespoons chopped parsley
2 tablespoons chopped rosemary
2 tablespoons chopped basil
2 tablespoons chopped cilantro
2 tablespoons chopped chives
1 cucumber, peeled and diced
1 red bell pepper, cut into strips
1 yellow bell pepper, cut into strips
½ cup halved cherry tomatoes
4 slices of red onion, separated into rings
¼ cup apple cider vinegar
2 tablespoons flaxseed oil
Juice of 2 limes
Juice of 1 lemon
1 pound grilled chicken breast, chilled and diced

Combine all the ingredients except the chicken in a large bowl and toss until evenly mixed. Arrange the chicken on top of the salad.

· Summer Confetti Salad ·

(SERVES 6)

10 Belgian endive leaves
1 avocado, cubed
1 cup cooked corn
½ cup diced red bell pepper
½ cup diced green bell pepper
Juice of 1 lemon
3 tablespoons avocado oil or sesame oil
Salt, to taste

Combine all the ingredients in a salad bowl. Drizzle with a dressing of lemon juice, avocado oil, and salt.

· Sweet 'n' Sour Cucumber and Red Onion Salad ·

(SERVES 4)

6 Kirby cucumbers, halved lengthwise, or 3 large, peeled
1 small red onion, quartered and sliced
4 plum tomatoes, quartered (optional)
2 tablespoons fresh lemon juice
2 tablespoons apple cider vinegar
Stevia Plus, to taste (see page 176)
Chopped dill weed, as desired
Chopped Italian (flat) parsley, as desired

Mix all the ingredients in a nonmetal container; cover. Refrigerate at least 6 hours, shaking the pan occasionally, to allow the flavors to develop.

· Marinated Vegetable Salad ·

This entire salad, with its dressing, is marinated in the refrigerator for several hours, or overnight.

(SERVES 8)

DRESSING:

½ cup flaxseed oil

⅓ cup apple cider vinegar

1 garlic clove (optional)

½ teaspoon dry mustard

1 teaspoon celery seed

Stevia Plus, to taste (see page 176)

2 tablespoons chopped Italian (flat) parsley

1 tablespoon chopped dillweed

SALAD:

2 cups cauliflower florets

4 carrots, sliced

4 stalks celery, chopped

2 cups shredded green cabbage

1 green bell pepper, cut into strips

1 red bell pepper, cut into strips

1 yellow bell pepper, cut into strips

1 (14-ounce) can artichoke hearts, rinsed, drained, and quartered

½ cup black olives, rinsed, drained, and halved

Cayenne, to taste
Salt, to taste
½ cup chopped dillweed
½ cup chopped Italian (flat) parsley
8 Italian (flat) parsley sprigs
8 dillweed sprigs

Combine the dressing ingredients in a blender or mini processor; blend well. Place all the vegetables and the olives, cayenne, salt, and chopped herbs in a flat nonmetal container with a lid. Pour the dressing over; place the lid on tightly and shake well. Refrigerate several hours or overnight to allow the flavors to develop, shaking occasionally. Adjust the seasonings if desired. Before serving, fold in 8 sprigs of Italian parsley and dillweed.

· *Shrimp Niçoise Salad* ·

(SERVES 4)

SALAD:
　8 cups torn mixed leafy greens (Boston, romaine, baby
　　spinach, etc.)
　4 scallions, sliced, or fresh chives
　2 cups fresh green beans, steamed and chilled
　4 hard-boiled eggs, quartered
　1 cup halved black olives
　1 cup halved cherry tomatoes
　1 pound medium fresh or frozen shrimp, peeled and deveined

DRESSING:
　¼ cup apple cider vinegar
　½ teaspoon dry mustard

½ teaspoon garlic powder
¼ teaspoon dried dillweed
Pinch salt
¼ cup flaxseed oil
Lemon wedges, for garnish

Decoratively arrange all the salad ingredients (except the shrimp) on a plate. Whisk together the dressing ingredients; drizzle over the salad. Top with the shrimp and garnish with the lemon wedges.

HINT: You can replace fresh or frozen shrimp with four (6-ounce) cans shrimp, rinsed and drained.

· Lovely Chicken Salad ·

(SERVES 4)

1 pound cooked chicken breast, cut into strips
½ cup diced celery
½ cup shredded raw red cabbage
¼ cup diced orange bell pepper
¼ cup diced red bell pepper
¼ cup diced yellow bell pepper
2 scallions, chopped
¼ cup Easy Homemade Mayonnaise (page 228) or Spectrum
    Naturals Organic Mayonnaise
1 tablespoon natural unheated honey
1 tablespoon fresh lemon juice
1 teaspoon celery seed
Salt, to taste (optional)
Large romaine or Boston lettuce leaves

Chopped Italian (flat) parsley
Chopped toasted pecans (page 239)

Toss together the chicken strips, celery, cabbage, bell peppers, and scallions in a large bowl. Combine the mayonnaise, honey, lemon juice, celery seed, and salt, if using, in a small bowl; mix well. Add the mayonnaise mixture to the chicken mixture, tossing gently to coat. Cover and chill for one hour. Arrange the chicken salad on lettuce-lined plates. Garnish with the parsley and toasted pecans.

· Thai Coleslaw ·

(SERVES 4)

DRESSING:

   6 tablespoons rice vinegar
   5 tablespoons flaxseed oil
   1 tablespoon toasted sesame oil
   5 tablespoons smooth, all-natural peanut butter
   3 tablespoons low-sodium, wheat-free tamari
   ½ teaspoon Stevia Plus, or to taste (see page 176)
   2 tablespoons minced ginger
   1½ tablespoons minced garlic

SALAD:

   5 cups thinly sliced green cabbage
   2 cups thinly sliced red cabbage
   2 cups shredded napa cabbage or bok choy
   2 red bell peppers, thinly sliced
   2 carrots, julienned
   6 scallions, chopped

½ cup chopped cilantro
Dash salt
Cayenne, to taste
2 tablespoons toasted sesame seeds, for garnish

· Toasting Nuts ·

To toast any nut to include as a tasty ingredient in Hot Times recipes, spread the nuts in a single layer on a cookie sheet and heat in the oven for 15 to 20 minutes at 250°F.

In a small bowl, whisk together all the dressing ingredients. Toss the vegetables in a large bowl. Add the dressing and mix well. Add the cilantro, salt, and cayenne to taste; toss again. Garnish with the toasted sesame seeds.

· "Pear-fect" Fall Salad ·

(SERVES 2)

VINAIGRETTE:

  1 tablespoon minced scallion
  3 tablespoons apple cider vinegar
  3 tablespoons almond oil
  2 teaspoons unsweetened cranberry juice concentrate
  1 tablespoon natural unheated honey
  Salt, to taste (optional)

1 cup green and red seedless grapes, halved
4 cups torn red and green leaf lettuce (or baby greens)
2 ripe pears (Bartlett, Bosc, Anjou, etc.), cored and sliced
2 tablespoons toasted sliced almonds (page 239)

Combine all the vinaigrette ingredients in a small bowl; whisk to combine. (Or place in a small container with a lid and shake until well blended.) In a salad bowl, combine the grapes and lettuce. Add the pears and vinaigrette; toss gently. Sprinkle with the almonds.

· Tabbouleh Salad ·

(SERVES 6)

1 cup finely chopped parsley
1 stalk celery, finely chopped
½ cup capers
½ cup finely chopped scallions
2 garlic cloves, minced
½ cup finely chopped basil
5 cups cooked bulgur
3 tablespoons fresh lemon juice
3 tablespoons olive oil
1½ tablespoons low-sodium, wheat-free tamari
⅛ teaspoon cayenne
6 leaves mint, finely chopped, for garnish

Combine the parsley, celery, capers, scallions, garlic, and basil in a large bowl. Add the bulgur. In a cup or small bowl, blend the lemon juice, oil, tamari, and cayenne. Toss with the grain and vegetables. Marinate for 30 minutes. Serve chilled, garnished with the mint.

· Moroccan Carrot Salad ·

(SERVES 6)

1 pound whole carrots, scrubbed and rinsed
1 garlic clove
4 cups water
½ teaspoon salt (optional)
½ teaspoon paprika
¼ teaspoon ground cumin
⅛ teaspoon cinnamon
¼ cup fresh lemon juice
2 tablespoons almond oil
1 tablespoon chopped parsley, for garnish

In a medium saucepan, place the carrots and garlic in the water. Bring to a boil and simmer for about 20 minutes. Discard the garlic. Cut the carrots into rounds. Combine the salt, paprika, cumin, cinnamon, lemon juice, and oil. Blend well and toss with the carrots. Garnish with the parsley.

· Orient Express Salad ·

(SERVES 6)

1 (1-pound) package soba noodles (buckwheat noodles)
8 cups water
1 (2.1-ounce) package sea palm fronds (optional)
1 cup grated carrots
1 (4 ounce) package firm tofu, cut into thin strips
1 cup finely chopped scallions

1 cup chopped red cabbage, cooked
½ cup slivered almonds
½ cup minced fresh cilantro
3 tablespoons almond oil
3 tablespoons brown rice vinegar
¼ teaspoon salt (optional)

Boil the noodles in the water. Drain and set aside. (If using sea palm fronds, prepare by first washing, soaking, and boiling until soft. Add to the noodles.) Add the carrots, tofu, scallions, cabbage, almonds, and cilantro to the noodles and toss. Drizzle with the oil and vinegar and add the salt, if using. Serve either warm or chilled.

· *Favorite Israeli Salad* ·

(SERVES 4)

1 large red bell pepper, diced
1 large green bell pepper, diced
2 cucumbers, peeled, seeded, and diced
4 plum tomatoes, diced
3 scallions, white and green parts, thinly sliced
½ cup chopped parsley
2 tablespoons fresh lemon juice
2 tablespoons olive oil
Salt (optional)
6 cups torn romaine leaves

In a large bowl, combine the bell peppers, cucumbers, tomatoes, scallions, and parsley. In a small bowl, whisk together the lemon juice, olive oil, and salt, if using. Pour the dressing over the salad and toss until all the ingredients are well combined. Refrigerate for at least 1 hour to allow the flavors to blend. Serve over the romaine leaves.

SIDE DISHES

· Spinach-Stuffed Portobello Mushrooms ·

(SERVES 4)

4 large portobello mushroom caps, stems removed, gills
   remaining
4 garlic cloves, minced
¼ cup finely chopped onion
¼ cup finely chopped red bell pepper
¼ cup finely chopped yellow bell pepper
1 (10-ounce) package frozen chopped spinach, defrosted and
   squeezed dry
1 tablespoon olive oil
¼ cup freshly grated Parmesan cheese (optional)
¼ cup wheat-free, yeast-free spelt bread crumbs (French
   Meadow HealthSeed Spelt)
1 tablespoon minced Italian (flat) parsley
Salt, to taste (optional)
Dash cayenne
Flaxseed oil

Preheat the oven to 375°F. Lightly coat a large baking pan with olive oil spray. Wipe the portobello caps well. In a medium skillet, sauté the garlic, onion, peppers, and spinach in the olive oil. Stir in the remaining ingredients (except the flaxseed oil), continuing to sauté for a few minutes more. Mound the stuffing on top of the mushrooms, pressing firmly.

Place on a baking pan; bake 15 minutes. Broil for 1 minute, or until golden brown. Arrange on a platter; drizzle with the flaxseed oil.

· Springtime Ratatouille ·

(SERVES 4 TO 6)

2 tablespoons olive oil
1 medium onion, chopped
5 garlic cloves, minced
1 green bell pepper, cut into chunks
1 red bell pepper, cut into chunks
1 yellow bell pepper, cut into chunks (optional)
1½ cups sliced mushrooms
1 cup sliced zucchini
1 cup sliced yellow squash
1 (14-ounce) can tomato purée (Muir Glen)
3 scallions, cut into 4-inch lengths, white parts cut in half
　　lengthwise
2 cups plum or cherry tomatoes, quartered
¼ cup minced cilantro
¼ cup minced basil
¼ cup minced Italian (flat) parsley
½ cup freshly grated Parmesan cheese (optional)

In a large skillet, heat 1 tablespoon of the oil over medium heat. Add the onion, garlic, peppers, and mushrooms; sauté until the vegetables are tender. Remove to a separate bowl. Heat the remaining table-

spoons of oil and sauté the zucchini and yellow squash until softened. Stir in the pepper mixture and tomato purée; cook over
medium-low heat for about 10 minutes. Stir in the scallions, plum
tomatoes, cilantro, basil, and parsley; simmer, stirring occasionally,
until heated through (5 to 10 minutes). Serve, passing grated Parmesan cheese separately, if using.

· Fresh Spinach Sauté ·

(SERVES 2)

1 tablespoon olive oil
4 garlic cloves, crushed
1 pound fresh spinach, washed and trimmed
Salt, to taste
Dash cayenne
Fresh lemon juice
2 tablespoons toasted pine nuts (page 239)

Heat the olive oil in a large skillet; sauté the garlic just until slightly
golden, being careful not to let it get darker. Add the spinach and
gently sauté until the leaves just begin to wilt and the spinach is
coated with olive oil and garlic, about 2 minutes. Remove from the
heat; toss with the salt and cayenne. Drizzle the spinach with fresh
lemon juice and toss gently with the toasted pine nuts.

· Walnut Miso Sauce ·

(MAKES 1 CUP)

1 cup chopped walnuts
3 tablespoons light miso
2 tablespoons rice vinegar
2 tablespoons Dijon mustard
3 tablespoons water

Blend all ingredients in a blender or food processor. This sauce tastes great with spinach.

· Spaghetti Squash with Vegetables and Spring Herbs ·

(SERVES 4)

2 tablespoons olive oil
4 garlic cloves, crushed
2 cups hot cooked spaghetti squash
2 scallions, thinly sliced, diagonally
¼ cup snow peas, sliced diagonally
¼ cup steamed diced carrots
¼ cup steamed green beans, sliced diagonally
2 teaspoons minced thyme
2 tablespoons minced Italian (flat) parsley
1 tablespoon snipped chives

Salt (optional)

Cayenne, to taste

Additional minced fresh herbs, for garnish

¼ cup freshly grated Parmesan cheese (optional)

Heat 1 tablespoon of the olive oil in a large skillet over medium heat. Stir in the garlic and sauté for 2 minutes, stirring constantly, until garlic begins to turn golden (be careful not to let the garlic get darker). Stir in the cooked spaghetti squash, remaining tablespoon olive oil, scallions, snow peas, carrots, green beans, thyme, parsley, and chives, cooking just until heated through. Season with the salt, if using, and cayenne to taste. Garnish with the additional minced fresh herbs. Serve, passing Parmesan separately, if using.

· Brown Rice with Parsley Nut Sauce ·

(SERVES 6)

1 cup water

1 tablespoon olive oil

1 tablespoon kuzu dissolved in 2 tablespoons water or 1
    tablespoon arrowroot

6 scallions, chopped

1 cup finely chopped parsley

½ cup chopped toasted cashew pieces

1 tablespoon low-sodium, wheat-free tamari

4 cups cooked brown rice, fluffed with a fork

In a medium saucepan, heat the water and oil over low heat. Add the kuzu and stir until thick. Add the scallions, parsley, nuts, and tamari. Serve over the rice.

· Molded Vegetable Gel ·

(SERVES 4)

6 cups chicken stock or fish stock
5 tablespoons agar flakes
½ teaspoon salt (optional)
1 carrot, cut into ½-inch slices
4 watercress sprigs
1 zucchini, cut into ½-inch slices
1 cup arame, soaked in water for 15 minutes (optional)

Bring the stock to a boil in a soup pot. Sprinkle in the agar flakes and salt, if using. Simmer until the agar is dissolved, about 8 to 10 minutes. Arrange the vegetables in a shallow Pyrex pan. Carefully pour the liquid over vegetables. Let set and serve chilled.

· Broccoli with Lemon Crumbs ·

(SERVES 4)

1 large bunch broccoli, cut into florets
2 slices wheat-free, yeast-free spelt bread (French Meadow
    HealthSeed Spelt)
Juice of ½ lemon
Grated zest of 1 lemon
Dash cayenne
Dash salt (optional)
Flaxseed oil

Steam the broccoli. Whirl the bread in a blender or food processor to make crumbs. Lightly coat a medium skillet with olive oil spray. Toast the crumbs in the skillet over medium heat. Add the lemon juice, zest, and cayenne. Working quickly, stir the mixture until the bread crumbs are "lemony" and toasted. Remove the bread crumbs from skillet; let cool to room temperature. Stir in the salt, if using. Place the steamed broccoli on a platter; drizzle with the flaxseed oil and sprinkle with the lemon bread crumbs.

· Warm Anchovy Sauce ·

(SERVES 6)

6 tablespoons extra-virgin olive oil
8 anchovy fillets, well-rinsed, drained, and chopped
8 garlic cloves, crushed

Heat the oil over medium-low heat. Remove from the heat and add the garlic. Let sit for about 10 minutes. Do not cook. Stir anchovies into mixture and keep warm. Use as a sauce over vegetables.

· Chilled Asparagus with Roasted Bell Pepper Sauce ·

(SERVES 4)

1 pound thin asparagus, trimmed and steamed
2 large red or yellow bell peppers, or 1 of each
¼ cup extra-virgin olive oil
1 garlic clove, minced

2 teaspoons Dijon mustard

1 tablespoon chopped Italian (flat) parsley

1½ teaspoons fresh lemon juice

¼ cup toasted pine nuts (see p. 239)

Arrange the steamed asparagus on a decorative platter; chill. Char the peppers in the broiler or over a gas flame until blackened. Place in a paper bag; let stand 10 to 15 minutes. Peel, seed, and chop coarsely. Place peppers, olive oil, garlic, mustard, parsley, and lemon juice in a blender and purée until smooth. Drizzle the sauce over the asparagus and sprinkle with the toasted pine nuts. Serve immediately or refrigerate up to 4 hours.

· Autumn Squash Soufflé ·

(SERVES 4)

1 large acorn squash, halved, seeds and pulp removed

2 baking apples, peeled and cored (such as Granny Smith)

2 eggs, separated

½ teaspoon grated lemon zest

Stevia Plus to taste (see page 176)

½ teaspoon cinnamon

½ teaspoon ginger

Preheat the oven to 350°F. Pierce the squash rind with a fork and place cut-side-down in ½-inch of water on a rimmed baking sheet. Place the apples on the baking sheet. Bake the apples for 25 to 30 minutes, or until softened. Bake the squash for 40 minutes, or until rind is soft. Beat the egg yolks. Place 2 cups of the cooked squash and the apples, lemon zest, stevia, and two beaten egg yolks in a food processor or blender; process until smooth. In a separate bowl, whip the egg whites until stiff peaks form; add the cinnamon and ginger. Remove the squash mixture to a large bowl. Fold the egg whites gently into the squash mixture.

Prepare a water bath by filling a 9 x 13-inch or a 9 x 9-inch baking dish with about 1½ inches of water; place in the oven. Lightly coat a 2½ quart ovenproof bowl with olive oil spray. Carefully pour the squash mixture into the prepared bowl and set the bowl in the water bath. Bake the soufflé for 40 minutes, or until set. Remove the bowl from the water bath. Serve immediately.

· Quinoa "Risotto" with Caramelized Onions ·

(SERVES 6 TO 8)

2 tablespoons olive oil
1 red bell pepper, diced
2 cups sweet onions, sliced very thin
Chicken broth or vegetable broth, as needed
Salt, to taste
1½ cups quinoa, rinsed and drained
2½ cups water
½ teaspoon salt

Heat 1 tablespoon of the oil in large nonstick skillet. Add the peppers and onions; cook over low heat, stirring frequently, until the peppers are soft and the onions are golden, about 25 minutes. (Add a little broth as needed to keep the onions from sticking to the pan.) Season with the salt; keep warm.

Heat the remaining tablespoon of oil in a large saucepan. Add the quinoa; cook over medium-high heat, stirring, until lightly browned, about 7 to 8 minutes. Add the 2½ cups water and the ½ teaspoon salt; bring to a boil. Cover tightly; simmer until water has been absorbed and quinoa is thoroughly cooked, about 15 minutes. Fluff with a fork; stir in the warm peppers and onions.

· Spaghetti Squash Pancakes ·

(SERVES 4)

2 cups cooked spaghetti squash
1 to 2 eggs
Ground cinnamon, to taste
Stevia Plus, to taste (see page 176)

In a medium bowl, combine the cooked spaghetti squash with the egg, cinnamon, and stevia. Heat a nonstick griddle pan that has been lightly coated with olive oil spray. Ladle the squash mixture into the pan in portions of about 2 tablespoons per pancake and cook until small bubbles form on the surface. Flip the pancakes over and continue cooking until almost "dry." Repeat with the remaining batter.

VARIATION: For a savory treat, replace the cinnamon and stevia with herbs such as minced fresh cilantro, parsley, basil, and oregano.

HINT: Great as a breakfast pancake too!

· Aegean Green Beans ·

(SERVES 4)

1 tablespoon olive oil
1 teaspoon black mustard seeds
4 garlic cloves, minced

2 teaspoons grated ginger
1 pound fresh green beans, trimmed, steamed, and chilled
1½ tablespoons tahini
2 tablespoons minced cilantro
1 tablespoon minced parsley
Cayenne, to taste
½ tablespoon fresh lemon juice
Salt, to taste (optional)

Heat the oil in a large skillet over medium heat. Carefully add the mustard seed. When the seeds start to pop (just a few seconds), stir in the garlic, sautéing until the garlic begins to turn golden (be careful not to let the garlic burn). Stir in the ginger; sauté for 1 minute. Stir in the green beans, tahini, cilantro, parsley, cayenne, lemon juice, and salt, if using, sautéing until the mixture is well combined. Simmer until the green beans are evenly heated, being careful not to overcook. Best served hot or at room temperature.

· Dilled Tofu Mustard ·

(MAKES ABOUT 1 CUP)

1 tofu cake
2 tablespoons fresh lemon juice
2 tablespoons Dijon mustard
2 tablespoons walnut or sesame oil
2 tablespoons minced dill weed
½ teaspoon salt (optional)

Combine all ingredients in a blender or food processor and purée until creamy. This makes a great sauce to drizzle over cooked vegetables, or to use as a tasty dip with artichokes or raw veggies.

· *Burdock Carrot Kimpira* ·

(SERVES 6)

1 tablespoon olive oil
1 teaspoon toasted sesame oil
4 medium carrots, scrubbed and cut into shavings
2 medium burdock roots, scrubbed and cut into shavings
½ teaspoon low-sodium, wheat-free tamari

Heat the olive and sesame oils in a heavy skillet. Sauté the carrot and burdock for a few minutes. Add the tamari.

· *Bok Choy in Ginger and Garlic Sauce* ·

(SERVES 6)

3 bunches bok choy, sliced into 1½-inch strips
2 tablespoons toasted sesame oil
2 garlic cloves, minced
2 teaspoons grated ginger
1 teaspoon kuzu, diluted in 1 tablespoon cold water
¼ cup low-sodium, wheat-free tamari

Sauté the bok choy in the oil with the garlic and ginger. Add the diluted kuzu and stir until thickened. Add the tamari.

· Mung Bean Dal ·

(SERVES 6)

1 tablespoon sesame oil
½ teaspoon cinnamon
½ teaspoon cumin
1 onion, minced
3 cups mung beans or chickpeas
1 strip kombu
12 cups water
¼ teaspoon salt (optional)
3 cups Basamti rice or brown rice, for serving
6 cilantro sprigs, for garnish
6 slices fresh lemon, for garnish

Heat the oil in a soup pot. Sauté the cinnamon, cumin, and onion. Add the beans, kombu, and water. Cook for 45 to 60 minutes. Add the salt, if using. Serve over basmati or brown rice, garnished with the cilantro and lemon slices.

· Hijiki Noodles ·

(SERVES 6)

1 (1-pound) package soba noodles (buckwheat noodles),
  cooked and drained
1 (2.1-ounce) package hijiki seaweed, soaked in water, rinsed,
  and cut into strips
1 cup grated carrots
1 cup chopped celery
1 cup minced parsley
½ cup minced scallions
1 garlic clove, minced
6 tablespoons extra-virgin olive oil

Combine all the ingredients, except the oil, in a large bowl. Toss with the oil. Let stand for thirty minutes before serving.

Recipe excerpted from A. L. Gittleman, Super Nutrition for Women *(New York: Bantam, 2004), with permission.*

· Surprising Sweet Potato Casserole ·

(SERVES 8)

FILLING:

2 eggs, separated
¼ teaspoon cream of tartar
2 cups mashed sweet potatoes
½ cup coconut milk
¼ cup butter, melted
¼ cup natural unheated honey

1 teaspoon cinnamon
½ teaspoon ginger
½ teaspoon nutmeg

TOPPING:

2 tablespoons butter, melted
¼ cup date sugar
¼ cup spelt flour
½ cup chopped pecans

Preheat the oven to 350°F. In a small bowl, whip the egg whites until stiff and glossy. Beat in the cream of tartar. Place the remaining filling ingredients in a large bowl, and beat with an electric mixer on high speed (or use a food processor) until light and fluffy. Gently fold the egg whites into filling. Pour into a 2-quart baking dish that has been lightly coated with olive oil spray.

In a small bowl, combine the topping ingredients. Crumble the topping over the surface of the filling. Bake 30 minutes. Reduce the temperature to 325°F and bake an additional 20 minutes, or until casserole is set.

ENTREES

· Sweet and Sour Tempeh ·

(SERVES 6)

¼ cup water
¼ cup low-sodium, wheat-free tamari
½ teaspoon ground coriander
1 garlic clove, minced

2 (8-ounce) packages tempeh, cut into 1-inch cubes
¼ cup arrowroot

Preheat the oven to 350°F. In a small bowl, mix the water, tamari, coriander, and garlic. Dip the tempeh into the mixture, then drain and coat with arrowroot. Bake for 20 minutes.

· Sweet and Sour Sauce ·

(MAKES ABOUT 1 CUP)

1 onion, finely chopped
1 tablespoon toasted sesame oil
1¼ cups water
2½ tablespoons barley malt (or rice malt)
4 tablespoons low-sodium, wheat-free tamari (or soy sauce)
1 tablespoon rice vinegar
1 tablespoon tahini
1 teaspoon grated ginger
2 scallions, finely chopped
2 teaspoons kuzu, diluted in 2 tablespoons cold water

Sauté the onion in the oil for 5 minutes. Add the water, malt, tamari, vinegar, tahini, ginger, and scallions. Bring to a boil. Thicken with the kuzu and serve over tempeh, tofu, chicken, or turkey.

· Spelt Pasta with Mushroom Lentil Sauce ·

(SERVES 6)

1 garlic clove, minced
½ onion, finely chopped
1 stalk celery, finely chopped
1 carrot, finely chopped
2 tablespoons extra-virgin olive oil
1½ pounds whole peeled tomatoes (fresh or canned)
1 cup mushrooms, coarsely sliced
1 cup cooked lentils, drained
¼ teaspoon salt (optional)
1 pound spelt pasta or whole-grain pasta, cooked and drained

Sauté the garlic, onion, celery, and carrots in the oil. Add the tomatoes and simmer for 20 minutes. Add the mushrooms and lentils and simmer 20 minutes longer. Add the salt, if using. Toss with the cooked pasta.

· Tempeh Chili ·

(SERVES 4 TO 6)

2 (8-ounce) packages tempeh
2 (14-ounce) cans organic diced tomatoes (Muir Glen)
1 medium onion, diced
3 to 4 stalks celery, diced
4 to 6 garlic cloves, minced
1 tablespoon cumin
1 teaspoon ground coriander

1 teaspoon oregano
¼ teaspoon garlic powder
⅛ teaspoon ground cloves
¼ teaspoon cayenne, or to taste
¼ teaspoon powdered jalapeño chili, or to taste
½ teaspoon salt (optional)
3 tablespoons apple cider vinegar
½ cup chopped cilantro
2 tablespoons dried parsley
½ to 1 cup vegetable broth
8 ounces mushrooms, diced
Dash Stevia Plus, if needed (see page 176)

Combine all the ingredients except the mushrooms in a large soup pot over medium heat. Bring to a boil; reduce the heat and simmer, covered, for about 45 minutes, or until the vegetables are fork-tender. Add the mushrooms and simmer an additional 10 minutes. Taste and adjust spices as needed. If the chili tastes too spicy or sour, add a dash of stevia.

· Tofu Ceviche ·

(SERVES 4)

Juice of 6 limes
1 garlic clove, minced
3 tablespoons minced parsley
3 tablespoons minced cilantro
½ teaspoon salt (optional)
½ pound tofu, cut into 1-inch slices
1 cup cherry tomatoes (optional)

2 onions, thinly sliced

2 avocados, halved

Mix the lime juice, garlic, parsley, cilantro, and salt, if using. Pour over the tofu slices and marinate for 30 minutes or more. Pour off the excess juice and add the tomatoes and onions. Mix and serve in the avocado halves.

· Wonderful Winter Stew ·

(SERVES 6)

1 tablespoon peanut oil

1 medium daikon radish, peeled and diced

2 carrots, peeled and chopped

1 rutabaga, peeled and diced

1 large parsnip, peeled and diced

1 onion, diced

1 large sweet potato, peeled and diced

1 cup dried porcini mushrooms soaked in 1½ cups water
    (reserve the water)

6½ cups vegetable broth or chicken broth

1 tablespoon grated ginger

6 to 8 roasted garlic cloves

1 tablespoon Chinese 5-spice powder

1 jalapeño pepper (membrane and seeds removed), minced

2 (8-ounce) packages tempeh, diced

2 tablespoons low-sodium, wheat-free tamari

1 tablespoon kuzu, diluted in 2 tablespoons cold water

3 scallions, chopped, for garnish

Heat the oil in a large skillet over medium heat. Sauté the daikon, carrots, rutabaga, parsnip, onion, and sweet potato. Stir in the mushrooms and soaking water. Reduce the heat and add the broth, ginger, garlic, 5-spice powder, jalapeño, and tempeh. Simmer, covered, until the vegetables are just fork-tender, 20 to 40 minutes. Add the tamari and kuzu; stir well. Garnish with the scallions.

· Blackened Red Snapper ·

(SERVES 6)

1 tablespoon paprika
½ teaspoon onion powder
1 teaspoon cayenne
½ teaspoon dried thyme
½ teaspoon dried oregano
½ teaspoon dried basil
½ teaspoon salt (optional)
6 (5-ounce) red snapper fillets, about 1 inch thick
5 tablespoons olive oil
6 lemon wedges, for garnish

Combine the spices, herbs, and salt, if using, on a platter. Place a cast-iron skillet over medium heat until very hot. Dip the red snapper in the oil and coat with the spice mixture. Place the fish in the hot skillet for 1 minute. Turn and char the other side. Remove from the pan. Serve garnished with the lemon wedges.

· Herb-Crusted Salmon Fillet ·

(SERVES 4)

MARINADE:

2 tablespoons apple cider vinegar

1 tablespoon olive oil

1 garlic clove, minced

½ teaspoon dry mustard or 1 teaspoon Dijon

4 teaspoons natural unheated honey

1 tablespoon fresh lemon juice

2 tablespoons chopped Italian (flat) parsley

1 tablespoon chopped dillweed

1 pound salmon fillet

Mixed greens or spinach leaves, for serving

Combine the marinade ingredients in a blender or mini food processor and pour into a large plastic bag with a zipper closure. Add the salmon fillet, turning to coat. Refrigerate at least 2 hours, turning occasionally.

Preheat the oven to 375°F. Lightly coat a 9 x 13-inch baking pan with olive oil spray. Place the salmon in the baking dish and cover with the marinade. Bake the salmon about 25 minutes, or until almost cooked through. Broil 1 to 2 minutes just until salmon flakes and a golden herb crust starts to form. (Watch carefully.) Serve hot or chilled over mixed greens or fresh spinach leaves.

· *Simple Salmon Patties* ·

(SERVES 4)

1 pound salmon fillet, cooked, or 1 pound canned salmon,
   drained well
½ medium sweet onion, minced
¼ cup minced celery
2 tablespoons minced dillweed
2 tablespoons minced Italian (flat) parsley
1 garlic clove, minced
1 tablespoon fresh lemon juice or fresh lime juice
2 eggs, beaten
2 teaspoons Dijon mustard
½ cup wheat-free, yeast-free spelt bread crumbs (French
   Meadow HealthSeed Spelt)

Preheat the oven to 350°F. Lightly coat a baking sheet with olive oil
cooking spray. In a large bowl, flake the salmon with a fork. Combine
with the remaining ingredients. Shape the mixture into 8 patties and
place the patties on a baking sheet. Bake for 20 to 25 minutes, or until nicely browned and cooked through. Freezes and reheats well.

· *Chicken Cacciatore* ·

(SERVES 4)

1 pound boneless, skinless chicken breast halves
Salt (optional)
1 tablespoon olive oil
1 large onion, coarsely chopped

1 cup dried porcini mushrooms, reconstituted in 1 cup hot
   water
1 medium green bell pepper, coarsely chopped
1 medium red bell pepper, coarsely chopped
1 cup sliced button mushrooms
5 garlic cloves, minced
1 (16-ounce) can organic tomatoes with purée (Muir Glen)
2 tablespoons dry white wine (organic and sulfite-free)
½ cup minced Italian (flat) parsley
2 teaspoons dried basil
1 teaspoon dried oregano
1 tablespoon kuzu, diluted in 2 tablespoons water
Hot cooked spaghetti squash, for serving

Season the chicken breasts lightly with the salt, if using. Heat the
olive oil in a large nonstick skillet over medium-high heat. Add the
chicken and sauté, turning once, until lightly browned, about 3 minutes. Remove the chicken and set aside. Add the onion to the skillet
with ½ cup of the porcini water. Cook, stirring occasionally, until the
onion is softened, about 2 to 3 minutes. Add the peppers, porcini
mushrooms, button mushrooms, and garlic and cook 3 minutes
longer. Add the tomatoes and stir, breaking up the tomatoes with a
spoon. Add the wine, parsley, basil, and oregano. Add the remaining
porcini water as needed. Cut the chicken into strips and return it to
the skillet, along with any pan juices that have collected. Reduce the
heat to medium-low and simmer, uncovered, stirring occasionally,
until the chicken is just cooked through, about 5 minutes. Stir the
kuzu into the chicken mixture, stirring until thickened. Serve over
the hot spaghetti squash.

HINT: You can double the recipe and freeze the leftover portions.

· Honey Lemon Chicken on the Grill ·

(SERVES 4)

MARINADE:

3 tablespoons natural unheated honey

2 garlic cloves, mashed

2 scallions, sliced

½ teaspoon coriander

¼ teaspoon ginger

Salt, to taste

⅛ teaspoon cayenne, or to taste

¼ cup fresh lemon juice

1½ teaspoons grated lemon zest

8 skinless chicken thighs

3 tablespoons chopped parsley

2 tablespoons chopped cilantro

1½ teaspoons grated lemon zest

Lemon slices, for garnish

Prepare the grill for medium-high heat. In a small bowl, whisk together the marinade ingredients. Pour the marinade into a plastic bag with a zipper closure. Add the thighs to the marinade and refrigerate for at least 30 minutes, shaking the bag occasionally to evenly distribute the marinade.

Place the thighs on the preheated grill. Grill the thighs for 20 minutes, brushing periodically with the marinade, until the thighs are thoroughly cooked and the juices run clear when the chicken is pierced with a fork. Sprinkle with the parsley and cilantro and the 1½ teaspoons lemon zest. Garnish with the lemon slices.

HINT: Serve with assorted grilled vegetables.

Variation: The chicken thighs can also be baked on a baking sheet (lightly coated with olive oil spray) in a 400°F oven. Bake about 30 minutes, brushing the chicken periodically with the marinade, until the thighs are thoroughly cooked and the juices run clear when the thighs are pierced with a fork.

· *Tangy Holiday Chicken* ·

(SERVES 6)

3 tablespoons sesame oil
½ teaspoon grated ginger
½ teaspoon coriander
½ teaspoon cardamom
½ teaspoon cumin
3 whole chicken breasts, skinned and halved
1 onion, sliced
2 carrots, sliced
1 cup cauliflower florets
1 cup green beans pieces, 1 inch long
2 cups water
¼ teaspoon salt (optional)
1 large butternut squash, cooked and puréed

Heat the oil in a skillet. Sauté the ginger, coriander, cardamom, and cumin in the oil. Add the chicken, onion, and carrots. Sauté until the chicken is golden and the onions are translucent. Add the cauliflower, green beans, water, and salt, if using. Cover and cook 15 more minutes. Add the puréed squash and cook 5 minutes longer.

· Pot Roast with Sweet Potatoes and Vegetables ·

(SERVES 8)

½ cup low-fat, low-sodium beef broth or stock
4 pounds boneless chuck roast or brisket
3 large onions, sliced
4 garlic cloves, sliced
Salt, to taste
Cayenne, to taste
½ cup organic crushed tomatoes (Muir Glen)
1 bay leaf
2 medium sweet potatoes, peeled and cut into chunks
4 medium carrots, peeled and cut into chunks
½ pound button mushrooms, quartered

Heat the beef broth in a Dutch oven. Braise the chuck roast or brisket until well browned on both sides; remove. Lay half of the sliced onions and garlic in the Dutch oven; place the meat on top. Season with the salt and cayenne. Place the remaining onions and garlic on top of the meat and add the crushed tomatoes and bay leaf and enough water to just reach the top of the meat. Bring to a boil, reduce heat to low; cover. Simmer about 2 hours (adding additional water as needed) or until meat starts to feel tender when pierced with a fork. Remove the meat; let cool slightly. Add the sweet potatoes, carrots, and mushrooms to the pot; place the meat on top of the vegetables; cover. Continue to simmer, adding small amounts of water as needed, for an additional 1 to 2 hours, or until the meat is tender enough to cut with a fork. Remove the meat; let rest 20 minutes;

slice thinly. Arrange the meat on a platter with the vegetables (remove bay leaf), passing the gravy separately.

CROCK-POT VARIATION: Rub the meat with salt and cayenne. Brown the meat in 1½ tablespoons olive oil in a heavy skillet; place in a Crock-Pot. Add ½ cup beef broth; cook on high for 3 hours. Add the vegetables, bay leaf, and crushed tomatoes (optional) and continue cooking on high for about 2 hours additional, or until meat is tender. Remove bay leaf.

HINT: For a rich aromatic gravy, purée half of the vegetables and gravy in a blender and stir into the remaining portion.

· Sassy Beef and Vegetable Kabobs ·

The beef is marinated for up to 4 hours before being
threaded on the skewers and grilled.

(SERVES 4)

MARINADE:

4 garlic cloves, crushed

2 scallions, chopped

1 tablespoon low-sodium, wheat-free tamari

1 tablespoon rice vinegar

1 tablespoon fresh lime juice

1 teaspoon tahini

1 teaspoon Dijon mustard

1 tablespoon rice bran oil

1½ tablespoons grated ginger

2 teaspoons toasted sesame seeds

KABOBS:

1 pound lean boneless beef sirloin, cut into 1½-inch cubes
1 onion, cut into chunks
1 green bell pepper, cut into chunks
1 red bell pepper, cut into chunks
1 large zucchini, cut into 1-inch slices
1 large yellow squash, cut into 1-inch slices
Cherry tomatoes
Button mushrooms

GLAZE:

¼ cup natural unheated honey
1 tablespoon low-sodium, wheat-free tamari

Prepare the grill for medium-high heat. Combine all the marinade ingredients in a plastic bag with a zipper closure. Add the beef and marinate for 2 to 4 hours, shaking the bag occasionally to distribute the marinade evenly. Drain the beef, reserving the marinade. Thread the beef and vegetables onto skewers.

Grill about 10 minutes, basting frequently with the reserved marinade and turning the skewers often to ensure even cooking. Mix the glaze ingredients together; baste the skewers and continue grilling for about 5 minutes or until the beef is cooked through and the vegetables are lightly charred.

HINT: Use half of the glaze for basting, reserving the remainder as a dipping sauce. (Do not use the remaining marinade for dipping unless it is boiled for 10 minutes.)

· *Hearty Hungarian Goulash* ·

(SERVES 6)

3 tablespoons olive oil
1 cup sliced onion
2½ pounds beef (chuck steak), cut into 2-inch strips
1 teaspoon paprika
¼ teaspoon salt (optional)
½ cup dry white wine
1 pound whole peeled tomatoes, fresh or canned

Preheat the oven to 350°F. Heat the olive oil in a large ovenproof skillet (with a lid) over medium heat. Sauté the onion and meat. When the onions are golden, add the paprika and salt, if using. Add the wine and cook a few minutes longer. Add the tomatoes, cover, and bake for 1½ hours. Check after 45 minutes and add a little water if necessary.

· *Middle Eastern Lamb Loaf* ·

(SERVES 4)

2 pounds ground lamb
4 garlic cloves, minced
1 medium onion, chopped
2 tablespoons minced red bell pepper
2 tablespoons minced green bell pepper
1 egg
¼ cup wheat-free, yeast-free spelt bread crumbs (French
    Meadow HealthSeed Spelt)
3 tablespoons chopped cilantro

3 tablespoons chopped parsley

2 teaspoons cumin

2 teaspoons coriander

2 teaspoons cinnamon

2 teaspoons chopped ginger

Preheat the oven to 375°F. Combine all the ingredients in a large bowl. Shape into a loaf. Place on a broiler pan that has been lightly coated with olive oil spray. Bake for 45 minutes, or until cooked through.

VARIATION: Place half the lamb mixture on the pan and cover with 1 (10-ounce) package frozen chopped spinach that has been defrosted and squeezed dry. Top with the other half of the lamb mixture, pressing firmly to seal. Bake as directed.

DESSERTS

· Strawberry Granita ·

(MAKES 6 SERVINGS)

3 teaspoons Stevia Plus or to taste, plus additional for sprinkling (see page 176)

½ cup water

1 pint hulled frozen strawberries

1½ teaspoons fresh lemon juice

6 whole strawberries, halved

Dissolve the 3 teaspoons stevia in the water. In a food processor, using a steel knife, process the frozen strawberries, lemon juice, and dissolved stevia until almost smooth. Pour into an 8 x 8-inch metal baking pan and cover with plastic wrap. Freeze until partly frozen, about 2 hours; stir with a fork to break up any ice crystals. Continue freezing for several hours or until completely frozen.

To serve, let the granita stand at room temperature about 10 minutes, or until slightly softened. Scrape into bowls using a spoon. Garnish with the strawberry halves sprinkled with Stevia Plus.

· *Banana Cheesecake in a Cup* ·

(SERVES 4)

1 cup large-curd cottage cheese
2 ripe bananas, frozen
¾ teaspoon vanilla extract
1 tablespoon natural unheated honey
4 teaspoons chopped toasted pecans
Cinnamon

Cream the cottage cheese in a blender or food processor. Add the frozen bananas, vanilla, and honey, processing just until bananas are incorporated. Divide into small bowls. Sprinkle with chopped pecans and cinnamon; serve immediately.

VARIATION: For a chocolate treat, add 2 teaspoons unsweetened cocoa to the banana mixture.

· Cool Caribbean Fruit Pops ·

(12 SERVINGS)

1 banana, peeled and cut into chunks
1 mango, peeled, pitted, and sliced
1 cup fresh pineapple chunks
⅓ cup strawberries, cleaned and hulled
2 kiwis, peeled and halved
½ cup unsweetened pineapple juice
½ cup coconut milk
¼ cup natural unheated honey
1 tablespoon fresh lime juice

Coarsely chop all the fruit and set aside about a third. In a food processor fitted with the steel knife (or a blender), combine the two-thirds of the chopped fruit with the pineapple juice, coconut milk, honey, and lime juice. Process until almost smooth; gently stir in the reserved chopped fruit. Spoon into popsicle molds, placing a wooden popsicle stick into each. Freeze until firm, several hours or overnight.

· Silky Swirled Pudding ·

(4 SERVINGS)

4 ounces silken tofu, drained
4 ounces firm tofu, drained (Mori-Nu brand is preferable)
1 tablespoon pure maple syrup
1 teaspoon vanilla extract
¼ teaspoon almond extract

2 tablespoons unsweetened raspberry preserves, mixed with
  ¼ teaspoon honey
2 tablespoons unsweetened apricot preserves, mixed with
  ¼ teaspoon honey
½ teaspoon Stevia Plus (see page 176)
½ teaspoon grated lime zest
2 tablespoons fresh raspberries, for garnish
2 tablespoons fresh blackberries, for garnish
2 tablespoons sliced fresh strawberries, for garnish

In a blender on high speed, whip the silken and firm tofu until smooth. Add the maple syrup and extracts and continue blending until thick and creamy. Using a small teaspoon, carefully swirl in the raspberry preserves with a backward motion. Repeat with the apricot preserves. Use the edge of the spoon to swirl the preserves throughout the pudding without mixing thoroughly. Add the stevia and lime zest and continue blending. Divide the pudding into glass bowls, garnish with the fresh berries, and serve immediately.

NOTE: As tofu continuously releases liquid, this recipe is not suitable for storing in the refrigerator to be served at a later time.

· *Mango Surprise* ·

(SERVES 4)

1½ cups water
1 tablespoon apple juice concentrate
3 tablespoons agar flakes
1½ cups mango pieces
2 teaspoons fresh lime juice

Bring the water and apple concentrate to a boil in a small saucepan. Add the agar flakes and simmer until dissolved, about 8 to 10 minutes. Let cool. Purée the mango and lime juice in a blender or food processor. Add to the cooled agar mixture and blend until smooth. Divide into serving cups and chill.

· Coconut Citrus Frozen Yogurt ·

(SERVES 6)

2 tablespoons kuzu
2 tablespoons fresh lime juice
2 tablespoons fresh lemon juice
½ cup natural unheated honey
½ cup coconut milk
1 teaspoon vanilla extract
1 teaspoon Stevia Plus (see page 176)
1 egg
Grated zest of 1 lemon
Grated zest of 1 lime
1 cup plain yogurt (low-fat or whole-milk)
½ cup unsweetened coconut

Dissolve the kuzu in the lime and lemon juices. In a saucepan over medium heat, mix the juice mixture, honey, coconut milk, vanilla, and stevia. Bring to a boil, stirring often. When the mixture thickens, remove from the heat; let cool slightly. In a small bowl, beat the egg with the lemon and lime zests. Return the juice mixture to low heat, stirring constantly. Slowly whisk in the egg mixture. Simmer, stirring constantly, for 2 minutes. Chill 10 minutes in the refrigerator. Fold in the yogurt and coconut. Pour into an ice cream machine and process according to the manufacturer's directions. Serve immediately.

VARIATION: Without an ice cream machine: After mixing the ingredients, place in a freezer-safe container with an airtight lid. Stir every hour for 3 to 4 hours until the mixture reaches the texture of sorbet.

HINT: The texture of this frozen yogurt is best when it is served immediately.

· *Refreshing Summer Fruits with Ricotta Dip* ·

(SERVES 4)

2 cups ricotta cheese (part-skim or whole-milk)
½ cup plain yogurt (low-fat or whole-milk)
1 tablespoon natural unheated honey
1 teaspoon vanilla extract
¼ teaspoon cinnamon, or to taste
4 cups fresh fruit, cut into chunks (pineapple, berries, melon, etc.)

Combine all the ingredients except the fruit in a blender or food processor; purée until smooth. Pour into a bowl and refrigerate until serving time. Arrange the fruit decoratively around a large plate and place the dip in the center.

· Berry Beautiful Meringues ·

(MAKES 8)

SHELLS:

   3 large egg whites
   ⅛ teaspoon salt
   ½ teaspoon cream of tartar
   ¼ teaspoon almond extract
   1 tablespoon natural unheated honey

GARNISH:

   1 cup heavy whipping cream
   1½ tablespoons natural unheated honey
   Cinnamon

FILLING:

   1 cup sliced fresh strawberries
   1 cup fresh raspberries
   1 cup fresh blackberries

Preheat the oven to 325°F. Line a baking sheet with baking parchment. With an electric mixer on high speed, beat the egg whites until foamy. Sprinkle the salt and cream of tartar evenly over the egg whites, add the almond extract, and beat until soft peaks form. Slowly drizzle the 1 tablespoon of honey over the egg whites, beating until stiff peaks form. Drop 8 portions of the meringue onto the parchment. With the back of a spoon, carefully smooth the centers while pushing toward the edge, forming a well. Bake 1 hour; turn oven off. Let cool in the oven with the door closed. Gently remove the meringues from the parchment.

Whip the cream and the 1½ tablespoons of honey to form stiff peaks. Carefully spoon the berries into the meringue shells. Top each with a dollop of whipped cream and sprinkle with cinnamon. Arrange on a decorative plate; serve immediately.

· Apple, Cranberry, and Pear Crisp ·

(8 SERVINGS)

FILLING:

2 baking apples, peeled, cored, and sliced (Granny Smith, Gala, etc.)

2 pears, peeled, cored, and sliced

½ cup fresh or frozen cranberries

1 tablespoon oat flour

½ teaspoons Stevia Plus (see page 176)

2 tablespoons fresh lemon juice

CRUST:

⅓ cup oat flour

1 scoop vanilla Fat Flush Whey Protein (see page 176)

1½ teaspoons Stevia Plus (see page 176)

½ to 1 teaspoon cinnamon

2 tablespoons butter, chilled

½ cup steel-cut oats, soaked in ½ cup hot water until softened

¼ cup chopped walnuts

Preheat the oven to 375°F. Coat an 8 x 8-inch baking dish with olive oil spray. In a medium bowl, mix the apples, pears, and cranberries. In a small bowl, combine the 1 tablespoon oat flour and the stevia. Stir in the lemon juice, mixing until the stevia is dissolved. Pour over the fruit and toss until well coated.

In a separate bowl, combine the ⅓ cup oat flour, whey protein, 1½ teaspoons stevia, and cinnamon. Cut in the butter, using a pastry blender or 2 knives, until only small lumps remain. Stir in the soaked oats. The oat flour mixture should resemble thick paste. (Stir in a small amount of additional water if needed.) Fold in the walnuts.

Pour the fruit mixture into the prepared pan and spread the crust mixture over the top. Bake 45 minutes, or until brown and crispy on top. For a pretty finish, place under the broiler for the last minute, watching carefully. Remove; let cool for 10 minutes before serving.

· Crunchy Flaxy Almond Apples ·

(SERVES 2)

2 apples, cut into wedges and cored
2 tablespoons milled flaxseed
2 tablespoons crushed toasted sliced almonds (page 239)
Stevia Plus, to taste (see page 176)
Cinnamon, to taste

Place all the ingredients in a plastic bag with a zipper closure; shake well, coating all the apples with the flaxseed mixture. Divide onto plates and serve.

· Delightful Pumpkin Pie ·

(SERVES 8)

CRUST:
½ cup almond meal
¼ cup almond flour

1 teaspoon Stevia Plus (see page 176)

1 egg

2 tablespoons butter, melted

FILLING:

¼ cup natural unheated honey

¼ cup pure maple syrup

¼ cup date sugar

12 ounces cream cheese, at room temperature

½ cup coconut milk

2 cups unsweetened canned pumpkin

2 eggs

½ teaspoon cinnamon

½ teaspoon ginger

¼ teaspoon nutmeg

¼ teaspoon mace

¼ teaspoon allspice

⅛ teaspoon cloves

1 teaspoon vanilla extract

Freshly whipped cream, for garnish (optional)

Preheat the oven to 350°F. In small bowl, combine the almond meal and almond flour with the stevia. Beat the egg with the melted butter and pour into the almond mixture; stir well. Press into a 9- or 10-inch pie plate. As mixture may be sticky, place a layer of plastic wrap over the mixture and press it into the pie plate. When the mixture is evenly pressed into the plate, discard the plastic. Bake the crust about 12 minutes, or until crust just starts to brown; let cool.

Fold the honey, maple syrup, and date sugar into the cream cheese. Add the coconut milk, pumpkin, and eggs. Stir in the spices and vanilla and mix until smooth. Pour the filling into the nut crust and bake for 1 hour, or until a toothpick inserted into the center of the pie comes out clean.

Let cool for 1 hour. (Pie can be served chilled, if desired.) Garnish with a dollop of whipped cream, if desired. Refrigerate leftover pie.

· Pears with Apricot-Grape Sauce ·

(2 SERVINGS)

½ cup chopped unsweetened dried apricots
½ cup halved red seedless grapes
1 tablespoon natural unheated honey
2 tablespoons water
2 medium ripe pears, cored
Cinnamon

Place the apricots, grapes, honey, and water in a small saucepan over medium heat; simmer, stirring constantly, until apricots soften. Slice the pears and arrange on plates in a fan shape. Drizzle the apricot-grape sauce evenly over each serving. Dust with cinnamon.

· Fresh Cranberry Sorbet ·

(6 SERVINGS)

2 cups fresh cranberries
¼ cup fresh orange juice
1 tablespoon grated orange zest
2½ cups water
¾ cup natural unheated honey
1 tablespoon fresh lemon juice
1 tablespoon kuzu

Place the cranberries, orange juice, zest, and ½ cup of the water in a medium saucepan; cook over medium heat until berries pop, 5 to 7 minutes. Coarsely mash the berries. Add the honey, lemon juice, kuzu, and remaining 2 cups of water. Simmer, stirring often, until the mixture forms into a syruplike consistency, about 1 hour.

Let cool. Pour into a freezer-safe container with an airtight lid. Freeze overnight.

The next day, stir with a fork periodically to keep ice crystals from forming. This sorbet will keep in the freezer for 2 to 3 weeks.

USING AN ICE CREAM MAKER: Pour the cooled cranberry mixture into the bowl of an ice cream maker; process according to the manufacturer's directions. Serve immediately or freeze.

· *Winter Fruits with Coconut Maple Sauce* ·

(6 SERVINGS)

2 cinnamon sticks
1 tablespoon kuzu, diluted in 2 tablespoons cold water
¼ cup natural unheated honey
1 cup coconut milk
1½ teaspoons maple extract
6 cups assorted fresh fruit
Cinnamon (optional)

In a medium saucepan, combine the cinnamon sticks, dissolved kuzu, and honey. Quickly stir in the coconut milk. Cook over medium heat, stirring constantly, until the mixture begins to boil and thicken slightly. Remove the cinnamon sticks. Remove the sauce from the heat; stir in the maple extract. Chill the sauce for at least 2 hours.

Alternate layers of fruits and sauce in parfait glasses or bowls.

Garnish with a sprinkle of cinnamon, if desired. Sauce may also be served warmed.

HINT: Fruits that go well with this sauce are apples, bananas, pears, grapefruit, grapes, pomegranates, and cranberries.

· Carrot Cake for a Crowd ·

(SERVES 15 TO 20)

1 cup spelt flour
1 cup oat flour
1 teaspoon non-aluminum baking powder
2 teaspoons baking soda
2 teaspoons cinnamon
1 teaspoon nutmeg
½ teaspoon salt
1 cup wheat germ
1 cup date sugar
1 tablespoon Stevia Plus (see page 176)
¼ cup natural unheated honey
¾ cup coconut oil (see Note) or rice bran oil
3 eggs, lightly beaten
1 teaspoon vanilla extract
2 cups shredded carrots
1 cup chopped walnuts
1 cup frozen chopped apples or pears, thawed and puréed
Lemon Honey Syrup (page 202)

Preheat the oven to 325°F. Coat a 9 x 13-inch pan with olive oil spray. In a large bowl, whisk together all the dry ingredients. Make a well in the center and add the honey, oil, eggs, and vanilla. Mix well; add the carrots, nuts, and puréed apples. (The batter will be very thick.) Spoon the batter into the cake pan, spreading evenly.

Bake 45 to 55 minutes, or until the center springs back when lightly tapped. Before the cake cools, poke all over with a fork; pour the Lemon Honey Syrup over top (quantity needed depends on amount of sweetness desired).

NOTE: Coconut oil is solid at room temperature. Place the jar in a bowl of hot water to bring the oil to a liquid state.

Conclusion

CONGRATULATIONS! BY READING THIS BOOK YOU HAVE taken the very first step toward understanding a nutritional approach to menopause. You have learned that menopause does not happen overnight. It is the culmination of years of lifestyle habits, both good and bad. You have read how heredity, smoking, diet, exercise, and stress all take their toll and contribute to the way in which the "change of life" affects you.

But it is never too late to change your habits—all it takes is your desire and commitment to assume responsibility for your own health. Step by step, one day at a time, you can begin to build, or even re-build, a sound foundation for a comfortable menopause and quality longevity.

Start simply by cutting back on sugar, coffee, artificial sweeteners, and saturated fat. Start adding the good oils to your diet. Use olive oil, sesame oil, macadamia nut oil, rice bran oil, and moderate amounts of coconut oil for cooking and baking. Experiment with the heart-healthy flaxseed oil for fresh salads or drizzling onto veggies or whole grains. Avoid margarine and vegetable shortening. For fiber and hard-to-come-by minerals, add more beans and sea vegetables to your menu plans.

Slowly increase your exercise. Begin walking regularly if you aren't currently doing it. Remember that walking, light aerobics, and weight training help to strengthen bone mass. Not only is exercise good for your body, it is also a great stress reliever.

Most of all, make this a special time of life for you. Take some quiet time for yourself on a daily basis. Meditation and deep breathing are excellent tools for calming the mind and smoothing out the ups and downs of modern-day living. Reading uplifting affirmations and spiritual books can often take you outside of yourself and renew your perspective on life. Treat yourself well and listen to your body/mind signals. Menopause can be a wonderful time for taking inventory of all aspects of your life. Explore this time with joy and adventure, because, for many women, the best is still ahead.

I hope this book will be as useful to you as researching it has been for me. It is comforting to know that the classic symptoms of menopause—night sweats, vaginal dryness, insomnia, and mood swings—are not inevitable. There are many vitamins, herbs, essential fatty acids, and homeopathic preparations that can help to balance a changing body chemistry—without side effects. I hope the recipe section that starts on page 195 will help you to turn the dietary recommendations discussed throughout the book into a delicious and nutritious reality.

Taking control of your menopause now will start you on a journey to continued health, vitality, and radiance. May your journey be blessed with happiness and wisdom as well.

RESOURCES

SPECIALTY SUPPLEMENTS, PRODUCTS, AND BOOKS

Uni Key Health Systems, Inc.
P.O. Box 2287
Hayden Lake, ID 83835
800-888-4353
www.unikeyhealth.com
208-762-9395 (fax)

To make shopping easier and more convenient, Uni Key Health Systems has distributed supplements to my clients and readers for nearly fifteen years. They offer self-health testing, including the salivary hormone kits mentioned in this book (pages 28, 149). Uni Key also carries the Fat Flush Whey Protein, a frequent ingredient in the Hot Times recipes, as well as my special Female Multiple, OsteoKey for strong bones, and hydrochloric acid to assist digestion. The Female Multiple is a copper-free multi with a unique 2:1 ratio of magnesium to calcium. It contains a full range of vitamins and minerals and 1000 mg of hesperidin complex for quelling hot flashes. Uni Key is a convenient source for other formulas, such as the Adrenal Formula and MenoCare and StressCare by Himalaya. Check out their Doulton water filter that I have personally used in my own home for over a decade. Visit them online or ask for a catalogue of their latest offerings and specials. If you can't find my books in the bookstore, Uni Key can send them to you directly.

French Meadow Bakery
2610 Lyndale Avenue South
Minneapolis, MN 55408
877-NO-YEAST
612-870-4740
www.womansbread.com
612-870-0907 (fax)

This company offers the highest-quality functional breads that are organic, dairy-free, yeast-free, oil-free, and sugar-free. Perfect for the diabetic, vegetarian, vegan, and individuals who keep kosher, Woman's Bread is a high-protein (7 g of protein per slice!), low-carb (7 g of carbs per slice!) bread that contains fermented soy isoflavones, flaxseeds, sprouted grains, and cranberries. The HealthSeed Spelt is a wheat-free, high-protein, sprouted bread rich in the omega-3 fatty acids. Look for French Meadow breads (including the Fat Flush Tortilla) in the refrigerated and frozen natural bread section in your local health food store or in specialty supermarkets.

www.annlouise.com
Feel free to visit my website for more information. On the site, current articles are available for your reading pleasure. And you are invited to drop by the Forum, an interactive messaging board that provides health- and nutrition-related support 24 hours a day, 7 days a week. You may also sign up to receive my free online e-letter, The Advisor.

WOMEN'S HEALTH INFORMATION

National Women's Health Network
514 10th Street NW, Suite 400
Washington, DC 20004
202-347-1140
www.nwhn.org
202-347-1168 (fax)

The network is a membership organization that works to advance women's health by advocating for a woman's right to decide about her reproductive health, creating a shift in the way menopause is viewed, and supporting a universal health care system.

National Women's Health Resource Center
157 Broad Street, Suite 315
Red Bank, NJ 07701
877-986-9472
www.healthywomen.org
732-530-3347 (fax)

This nonprofit organization is dedicated to helping women make informed decisions about their health and encouraging women to embrace healthy lifestyles to promote wellness and prevent disease.

Natural Woman Institute
8539 Sunset Boulevard
Los Angeles, CA 90069
888-489-6626
http://naturalwoman.org

The Natural Woman Institute seeks to educate women and their health care providers about natural alternatives for menopause therapy and supports research in the development of safe, effective natural hormone therapies. It offers referral lists of doctors who prescribe natural hormones and compounding pharmacies.

Society for Women's Health Research
1025 Connecticut Avenue NW, Suite 701
Washington, DC 20036
202-223-8224
www.womens-health.org
202-833-3472 (fax)

The society is the nation's only nonprofit advocacy group whose sole mission is to improve the health of women through research.

Office of Women's Health
Food and Drug Administration (FDA)
5600 Fishers Lane
Rockville, MD 20857
888-463-6332
www.fda.gov/womens

Established in 1994 within the U.S. FDA, the Office of Women's Health funds research and education on pressing women's issues and encourages participation of women in clinical studies. Its website provides information on current studies and the latest research results.

MENOPAUSE INFORMATION

Association of Reproductive Health Professionals
2401 Pennsylvania Avenue NW, Suite 350
Washington, DC 20037-1718
202-466-3825
www.arhp.org
202-466-3826 (fax)

The association is a professional membership organization for health care providers and others. It provides a number of brochures and online information for patients/consumers regarding birth control, osteoporosis, and other aspects of reproductive and women's medicine.

American Menopause Foundation, Inc.
The Empire State Building
350 Fifth Avenue, Suite 2822
New York, NY 10118
212-714-2398

www.americanmenopause.org
212-714-1252 (fax)

The American Menopause Foundation is the only independent, not-for-profit organization dedicated to providing support and assistance on all issues concerning the change of life. The network of volunteer support groups serves as a resource for women, families, organizations, and corporations. The foundation's newsletter, literature, and educational programs provide the latest information on scientific research and other pertinent facts.

North American Menopause Society

P.O. Box 94527
Cleveland, OH 44101
800-774-5342
www.menopause.org
440-442-2660 (fax)

The North American Menopause Society is a scientific nonprofit organization devoted to promoting women's health during midlife and beyond through understanding menopause. In addition to information about menopause, the organization offers a free monthly newsletter, a physician referral list, and a list of menopause discussion/support groups.

HormoneWise e-Digest

www.ssellman.com

Dr. Sherrill Sellman, N.D., created the Wise Woman site as a safe haven for women of all ages who seek information, education, resources, support, and holistic approaches to regain and maintain hormonal balance.

Power Surge

http://members.aol.com/dearest/intro.htm

Power Surge is a support network and online community for women in varying stages of menopause. Its purpose is to provide information and encourage discourse, enabling every woman to educate herself on the best method of treatment for her. Celebrated guest authors, physicians, naturopaths, psychotherapists, and nutritionists join in online conferences on a weekly basis.

Prime Plus

Red Hot Mamas Menopause Management Education Programs
23 North Valley Road

Ridgefield, CT 06877
203-431-3902
www.redhotmamas.org
203-894-1369 (fax)

Red Hot Mamas programs are sponsored at no charge by hospitals and health care providers throughout the United States. The website offers a community bulletin board, a monthly newsletter dedicated to providing the very latest information on menopause, and a list of local venues for educational programs and support groups.

BREAST CANCER INFORMATION

FORCE: Facing Our Risk of Cancer Empowered
934 North University Drive, PMB #213
Coral Springs, FL 33071
954-255-8732
www.facingourrisk.org

The FORCE website offers a chat room and resources for women at high risk for breast and ovarian cancer.

Mamm magazine
54 West 22nd Street, 4th Floor
New York, NY 10010
888-901-MAMM
www.mamm.com

Mamm is a magazine for women diagnosed with breast and reproductive cancers.

National Breast Cancer Coalition
1101 17th Street NW, Suite 1300
Washington, DC 20036
800-622-2838
www.natlbcc.org
202-265-6854 (fax)

The coalition is the nation's largest advocacy group for those with breast cancer. It trains individuals to be effective activists and to influence public policy, with the goal of ending breast cancer.

OSTEOPOROSIS INFORMATION

National Osteoporosis Foundation
1232 22nd Street NW
Washington, DC 20037
202-223-2226
www.nof.org

The National Osteoporosis Foundation is the leading nonprofit health organization dedicated to promoting lifelong bone health, while supporting research, education, and advocacy to find a cure for osteoporosis.

ESSENTIAL FATS INFORMATION

www.fatsforhealth.com
FATSforHEALTH.com brings you the latest news and information on omega-3 and omega-6 EFA supplements.

www.omega3ri.org
The Omega-3 Research Institute, Inc., is an independent, not-for-profit corporation devoted to facilitation of research, communication, and education on omega-3 polyunsaturated fatty acids.

www.omega-3info.com
Keep up with the latest details on omega-3 news by visiting the Omega-3 Information Service.

www.wisc.edu/fri/clarefs.htm
A great site at the University of Wisconsin, listing articles in medical journals . . . all about conjugated linoleic acid.

www.flaxcouncil.ca
This is the official website of the Flax Council of Canada, with everything from the latest research results to tasty recipes using this healthful plant.

HORMONE TESTING

Aeron LifeCycles Clinical Laboratory
1933 Davis Street, Suite 310
San Leandro, CA 94577
800-631-7900
www.aeron.com
510-729-0383 (fax)

BodyBalance
63 Zillicoa Street
Asheville, NC 28801
888-891-3061
www.bodybalance.com
828-253-4646 (fax)

Meridian Valley Clinical Laboratories
515 West Harrison
Kent, WA 98032
800-234-6825

Metametrix Clinical Laboratory
4855 Peachtree Industrial Boulevard, Suite 201
Norcross, GA 30092
800-221-4640
www.metametrix.com
770-441-2237 (fax)

Uni Key Health Systems
P.O. Box 2287
Hayden Lake, ID 83835
800-888-4353
www.unikeyhealth.com
208-762-9395 (fax)

ZRT Laboratory
1815 NW 169th Place, Suite 5050
Beverton, OR 97006
503-466-2445
www.salivatest.com
503-466-1636

Holistic Health Education

Clayton College of Natural Health
2140 11th Avenue South, Suite 305
Birmingham, AL 35205
800-995-4590
www.ccnh.edu
205-323-8232 (fax)

Established in 1980, Clayton is the world's leading college of natural health and holistic nutrition, with both degreed and certificate programs. It is accredited by the American Naturopathic Medical Certification and Accreditation Board and the American Association of Drugless Practitioners.

Referrals

For a referral to a medical doctor or osteopath who is knowledgeable in the use of natural hormone replacement, you can contact:

American College for Advancement in Medicine (ACAM)
23121 Verdugo Drive, Suite 204
Laguna Hills, CA 92653
800-532-3688
www.acam.com
949-455-9679 (fax)

The college is a not-for-profit medical society dedicated to educating physicians and other health care providers on the latest findings in preventive/nutritional medicine.

Naturopathic physicians are licensed in the following states: Alaska, Arizona, Connecticut, Hawaii, Maine, Montana, New Hampshire, Oregon, Utah, Vermont, and Washington and the District of Columbia. For a referral to a naturopathic physician who can guide you with natural hormone therapy, you can contact:

The American Association of Naturopathic Physicians
3201 New Mexico Avenue NW, Suite 350
Washington, DC 20016
866-538-2267
202-895-1392
www.naturopathic.org
202-274-1992 (fax)

To locate an osteopathic physician, practitioners who take a preventive approach to medical practice and emphasize the *whole person,* contact:

American Osteopathic Association
142 East Ontario Street
Chicago, IL 60611
800-621-1773
www.osteopathic.org
312-202-8200 (fax)

While most pharmacists fill prescriptions by simply filling bottles with premixed liquids or tablets, some still compound natural prescriptions individualized for your condition. To locate a compounding pharmacy near you, contact:

International Academy of Compounding Pharmacists (IACP)
P.O. Box 1365
Sugarland, TX 77487
800-927-4227
www.iacprx.org
713-495-0602 (fax)

Professional Compounding Centers of America, Inc. (PCCA)
9901 South Wilcrest Drive
Houston, TX 77099
800-331-2498
www.pccarx.com
800-874-5760 (fax)

GENERAL RESOURCES

The following list includes people and/or organizations whose philosophies are compatible with what I have outlined in *Hot Times*:

Health Research Institute and Pfeiffer Treatment Center
4575 Weaver Parkway
Warrenville, IL 60555-4039
630-505-0300
www.hriptc.org
630-836-0667 (fax)

Broda O. Barnes Research Foundation, Inc.
P.O. Box 110098
Trumbull, CT 06611
203-261-2101
www.brodabarnes.org
203-261-3017 (fax)

The American Holistic Medical Association
12101 Menaul Boulevard NE, Suite C
Albuquerque, NM 87112
505-292-7788
www.holisticmedicine.org
505-293-7582 (fax)

REFERENCES

CHAPTER ONE

Bartlik B, Goldstein MZ. "Maintaining Sexual Health After Menopause." *Psychiatr Serv* 51:751, 2000.

Million Women Study Collaborators. "Breast Cancer and Hormone-Replacement Therapy in the Million Women Study." *Lancet* 362:419, 2003.

Redwine L, et al. "Effects of Sleep and Sleep Deprivation on Interleukin-6, Growth Hormone, Cortisol, and Melatonin Levels in Humans." *J Clin Endocrinol Metab* 85:3597, 2000.

Shumaker SA, et al. "Estrogen Plus Progestin and the Incidence of Dementia and Mild Cognitive Impairment in Postmenopausal Women: The Women's Health Initiative Memory Study: A Randomized Controlled Trial." *JAMA* 289:2651, 2003.

Tworoger SS, et al. "Effects of a Yearlong Moderate-Intensity Exercise and a Stretching Intervention on Sleep Quality in Postmenopausal Women." *Sleep* 26:830, 2003.

Writing Group for the Women's Health Initiative Investigators. "Risks and Benefits of Estrogen Plus Progestin in Healthy Postmenopausal Women." *JAMA* 288:321, 2002.

Wurtman J. "Weight Gain at Menopause." *A Friend Indeed* 9(4):1, 1992.

CHAPTER THREE

Abraham GE, Grewal H. "A Total Dietary Program Emphasizing Magnesium Instead of Calcium: Effect on the Mineral Density of Calcaneus Bone in Postmenopausal Women on Hormonal Therapy." *J Repro Med* 35:503, 1990.

Bierennbaum ML, et al. "The Effect of Dietary Calcium Supplementation on Blood Pressure and Serum Lipid Levels, Preliminary Report." *Nutr Rep Int* 36:1147, 1987.

Bland J. "Building Stronger Bones." *Delicious* July/August:12, 1988.

Bouckaert JS, Said AH. "Fracture Healing by Vitamin K." *Nature* 185:849, 1960.

Burckhardt P, Michel CH. "The Peak Bone Mass Concept." *Clin Rheumatol* 8 (Suppl. 2):16, 1989.

Chapuy MC, Arlot ME. "Vitamin D3 and Calcium to Prevent Hip Fractures in Elderly Women." *N Engl J Med* 327:1637, 1992.

Daksky GP, et al. "Weight-Bearing Exercise Training and Lumbar Bone Mineral Content in Postmenopausal Women." *Ann Intern Med* 108:824, 1988.

Holden JM, Wolf WR, Merta W. "Zinc and Copper in Self-Selected Diets." *J Am Diet Assoc* 75:23, 1979.

Hollingberg P, Massey L. "Effect of Dietary Caffeine and Sucrose on Urinary Calcium Excretion in Adolescents." *Fed Protocol* 45:375, 1968.

Johnston CC, Longcope C. Editorial: "Premenopausal Bone Loss." *N Engl J Med* 323:1271, 1990.

Johnson NE, Smith EL, Freudenheirn JL. "Effects on Blood Pressure of Calcium Supplementation of Women." *Am J Clin Nutr* 42:12, 1985.

Lakshmanan FL, et al. "Calcium and Phosphorus Intakes, Balances, and Blood Levels of Adults Consuming Self-Selected Diets." *Am J Clin Nutr* 40:1368, 1984.

Lindsay R, et al. "Bone Response to Termination of Oestrogen Treatment." *Lancet* 1:1325, 1978.

McCarron DA, Morris CD. "Blood Pressure Response to Oral Calcium in Persons with Mild to Moderate Hypertension: A Randomized Double-Blind Placebo-Controlled Crossover Trial." *Ann Intern Med* 103:825, 1985.

Nielsen F, et al. "Effect of Dietary Boron on Mineral, Estrogen, and Testosterone Metabolism in Postmenopausal Women." *FASEB J* 1:394, 1987.

Oski FA. *Don't Drink Your Milk.* Syracuse, NY: Monica Press, 1983, p. 60.

Paganini-Hill A, et al. "Exercise and Other Factors in the Prevention of Hip Fracture: The Leisure World Study." *Epidemiology* 2:16, 1991.

Raloff J. "New Misgivings About Low Magnesium." *Sci News* 133:356, 1988.

Robert D, et al. "Hypercalciuria During Experimental Vitamin K Deficiency in the Rat." *Calcif Tissue Int* 37:143, 1985.

Spenser H, et al. "Effects of Small Doses of Aluminum-Containing Antacids on Calcium and Phosphorus Metabolism." *Am J Clin Nutr* 36:32, 1982.

Vieth R. "Vitamin D Supplementation, 25-Hydroxyvitamin D Concentrations, and Safety." *Am J Clin Nutr* 69:842, 1999.

Wenlock RW, Buss DH, Dixon EJ. "Trace Nutrients. 2. Manganese in British Food." *Br J Nutr* 41:253, 1979.

CHAPTER FOUR

Erlinger TP, et al. "Inflammation Modifies the Effects of a Reduced-Fat Low-Cholesterol Diet on Lipids: Results from the DASH-Sodium Trial." *Circulation* 108:150, 2003.

"Magnesium for Acute Myocardial Infarctions?" *Lancet* 338:667, 1991.

Marcuccio E, et al. "A Survey of Attitudes and Experiences of Women with Heart Disease." *Womens Health Issues* 13:23, 2003.

Press R, et al. "The Effect of Chromium Picolinate on Serum Cholesterol and Apolipoprotein Fractions in Human Subjects." *West J Med* 152(1):41, 1990.

Ridker PM, et al. "Comparison of C-Reactive Protein and Low-Density Lipoprotein Cholesterol Levels in the Prediction of First Cardiovascular Events." *N Engl J Med* 347:1557, 2002.

Simonoff M. "Chromium Deficiency and Cardiovascular Risk." *Cardiovasc Res* 18:591, 1984.

Singh RB, et al. "Can Dietary Magnesium Modulate Blood Lipids?" *J Am Coll Nutr* 9:527 (Abstract 23), 1990.

Taylor CB. "Spontaneously Occurring Angiotoxic Derivatives of Cholesterol." *Am J Clin Nutr* 32:40, 1979.

Vinson J, et al. "Beneficial Effects of Antioxidant Vitamins on Lipids and Lipid Peroxidation." *J Am Coll Nutr* 9:537 (Abstract 55), 1990.

CHAPTER FIVE

Christ-Crain M, et al. "Elevated C-Reactive Protein and Homocysteine Values: Cardiovascular Risk Factors in Hypothyroidism?: A Cross-Sectional and a Double-Blind, Placebo-Controlled Trial." *Atherosclerosis* 166:379, 2003.

Holmberg L, Anderson H. "HABITS (Hormonal Replacement Therapy After Breast Cancer—Is It Safe?), A Randomised Comparison: Trial Stopped." *Lancet* 363:453, 2004.

Klein V, et al. "Low Alpha-Linolenic Acid Content of Adipose Breast Tissue Is Associated with an Increased Risk of Breast Cancer." *Eur J Cancer* 36:335, 2000.

Writing Group for the Women's Health Initiative Investigators. "Risks and Benefits of Estrogen Plus Progestin in Healthy Postmenopausal Women." *JAMA* 288:321, 2002.

INDEX